Neuroscience Research Progress

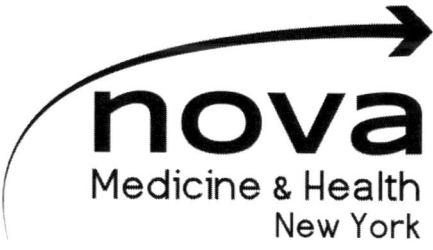

Neuroscience Research Progress

An Insight into Neuromodulation: Current Trends and Future Challenges
Natalia Arias (Editor)
Ana María Jiménez García (Editor)
2024. ISBN: 979-8-89113-445-4 (Hardcover)
2024. ISBN: 979-8-89113-531-4 (eBook)

Dendritic Spines: An Update
Ignacio González-Burgos, PhD (Editor)
2023. ISBN: 979-8-89113-080-7 (Hardcover)
2023. ISBN: 979-8-89113-138-5 (eBook)

Reticular Concept of Nervous System Physiology
Oleg Sotnikov, PhD (Editor)
2022. ISBN: 978-1-68507-996-3 (Hardcover)
2022. ISBN: 979-8-88697-350-1 (eBook)

Neuroscience and Technology Transform the Educational Ecosystem
Franco F. Orsucci (Editor)
Nicoletta Sala (Editor)
2022. ISBN: 979-8-88697-157-6 (Hardcover)
2022. ISBN: 979-8-88697-248-1 (eBook)

New Perspectives in Neuroscience
Prachi Srivastava, PhD (Editor)
Neha Srivastava, PhD (Editor)
Prekshi Garg (Editor)
2022. ISBN: 978-1-68507-754-9 (Softcover)
2022. ISBN: 978-1-68507-847-8 (eBook)

More information about this series can be found at
https://novapublishers.com/product-category/series/neuroscience-research-progress/

Leticia Granados-Rojas
Carmen Rubio
Editors

The Ketogenic Diet Reexamined

Myth vs. Reality

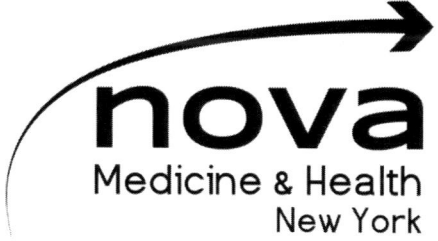

Copyright © 2024 by Nova Science Publishers, Inc.
DOI: https://doi.org/10.52305/KSTQ4025

All rights reserved. No part of this book may be reproduced, stored in a retrieval system or transmitted in any form or by any means: electronic, electrostatic, magnetic, tape, mechanical photocopying, recording or otherwise without the written permission of the Publisher.

We have partnered with Copyright Clearance Center to make it easy for you to obtain permissions to reuse content from this publication. Please visit copyright.com and search by Title, ISBN, or ISSN.

For further questions about using the service on copyright.com, please contact:

Copyright Clearance Center
Phone: +1-(978) 750-8400   Fax: +1-(978) 750-4470   E-mail: info@copyright.com

NOTICE TO THE READER

The Publisher has taken reasonable care in the preparation of this book but makes no expressed or implied warranty of any kind and assumes no responsibility for any errors or omissions. No liability is assumed for incidental or consequential damages in connection with or arising out of information contained in this book. The Publisher shall not be liable for any special, consequential, or exemplary damages resulting, in whole or in part, from the readers' use of, or reliance upon, this material. Any parts of this book based on government reports are so indicated and copyright is claimed for those parts to the extent applicable to compilations of such works.

Independent verification should be sought for any data, advice or recommendations contained in this book. In addition, no responsibility is assumed by the Publisher for any injury and/or damage to persons or property arising from any methods, products, instructions, ideas or otherwise contained in this publication.

This publication is designed to provide accurate and authoritative information with regards to the subject matter covered herein. It is sold with the clear understanding that the Publisher is not engaged in rendering legal or any other professional services. If legal or any other expert assistance is required, the services of a competent person should be sought. FROM A DECLARATION OF PARTICIPANTS JOINTLY ADOPTED BY A COMMITTEE OF THE AMERICAN BAR ASSOCIATION AND A COMMITTEE OF PUBLISHERS.

Library of Congress Cataloging-in-Publication Data

Names: Granados-Rojas, Leticia, editor. | Rubio, Carmen (Neurologist), editor.
Title: The ketogenic diet reexamined : myth vs. reality / editors Leticia Granados-Rojas, PhD, Researcher in Medical Sciences, Laboratory of Neuroscience II, National Institute of Pediatrics, Mexico City, Mexico, Carmen Rubio, PhD, in Medical Sciences, Neurophysiology Department, National Institute of Neurology and Neurosurgery, Mexico City, Mexico.
Description: New York : Nova Science Publishers, [2024] | Series: Neuroscience research progress | Includes bibliographical references and index. |
Identifiers: LCCN 2024009514 (print) | LCCN 2024009515 (ebook) | ISBN 9798891135437 (paperback) | ISBN 9798891136496 (adobe pdf)
Subjects: LCSH: Ketogenic diet. | Brain--Diseases--Diet therapy. | Nervous system--Diseases--Diet therapy.
Classification: LCC RC374.K46 K53 2024 (print) | LCC RC374.K46 (ebook) | DDC 616.8/04654--dc23/eng/20240313
LC record available at https://lccn.loc.gov/2024009514
LC ebook record available at https://lccn.loc.gov/2024009515

Published by Nova Science Publishers, Inc. † New York

Contents

Preface vii

Acknowledgments ix

Chapter 1 **The Molecular Mechanisms of the Ketogenic Diet in Epilepsy** 1
Moisés Rubio-Osornio, Rudy Luna,
Tarsila Elizabeth Juárez-Zepeda,
Leticia Granados-Rojas and Carmen Rubio

Chapter 2 **The Role of the Ketogenic Diet on Parkinson's Disease Symptoms** 23
Joyce Graciela Martínez-Galindo,
Ana Vigil-Martínez and Ernesto Ochoa

Chapter 3 **The Ketogenic Diet and Alzheimer's Disease** 41
Ernesto Ochoa, Fernando Gatica, Zayra Morales,
Héctor Romo-Parra,
Luis Antonio Marín-Castañeda and Carmen Rubio

Chapter 4 **The Ketogenic Diet in Neuropsychiatric Disorders** 61
Tarsila Elizabeth Juárez-Zepeda, Carmen Rubio,
Diana Molina-Valdespino,
Luis Antonio Marín-Castañeda
America Vanoye Carlo and Leticia Granados-Rojas

Chapter 5 **The Ketogenic Diet and Cancer Prevention** 93
Fernando Gatica, Noél Gallardo, Eric Uribe,
Diana Flores, Vanessa Mena, Amalia Alejo,
David Vázquez and Carmen Rubio

Chapter 6	**The Ketogenic Diet and Neuroglia**..............................119 Eric Uribe, Carmen Rubio, Vanessa Mena, Noel Gallardo, Diana Flores, David Vázquez and Moisés Rubio-Osornio	
Chapter 7	**The Regional Expression of NKCC1 Cotransporter in the Dentate Gyrus of Rats Fed with a Ketogenic Diet**......................................141 Karina Jerónimo-Cruz, Tarsila Elizabeth Juárez-Zepeda, Joyce Graciela Martínez-Galindo, Miguel Tapia-Rodríguez, America Vanoye Carlo and Leticia Granados-Rojas	
Index	157	

Preface

Ketogenic diet (KD) is rich in fat, low in carbohydrates and adequate in protein. Its name derives from the fact that it increases ketone bodies that induce a state of ketosis where cells use ketone bodies as an alternative energy substrate. The diet was initially used as an effective non-pharmacological treatment for refractory epilepsy with beneficial results. However, in recent years this diet has proven to be useful in the treatment of other neurodegenerative diseases, such as Alzheimer's and Parkinson's diseases. In addition, KD has shown to be immensely beneficial in the treatment of some neuropsychiatric disorders such as schizophrenia, autism spectrum disorder, depression, anxiety and bipolar disorder as well as in the management of cancer. This book summarizes the researches on advances on the most effective methods or ways of KD administration. And on its effects on the treatment of the diseases or disorders as those mention above. Also, special emphasis is laid on the cellular and molecular mechanisms behind the curative effects of the diet in each of the diseased conditons.

This book will invariably be of benefit to students in any academic level and discipline, researchers in various disciplines and, in general, anyone interested in the subject. It is intended to raise awareness in the general public about on the usefulness of ketogenic diet as an adjunct therapy for the treatment of different brain diseases and metabolic problems.

Finally, researches in this field in recent years have all pointed out the favorable impact of KD on neurological and neuropsychiatric diseases, and on cancer. However, it is needed large and well-designed randomized clinical trials to determine the safety and efficacy of ketogenic diet, based on long-term data, in the treatment of patients with these diseases.

Leticia Granados Rojas,
Researcher in Medical Sciences, National Institute of Pediatrics, Mexico

Carmen Rubio,
Researcher in Medical Sciences, National Institute of Neurology and Neurosurgery, Mexico

Acknowledgments

We express our profound gratitude to all authors for their invaluable contribution to each chapter of this book. Our thanks also go to Nova Science Publishers for its support and facilities for the consolidation of this book; and finally, to the English language editing team.

Leticia Granados-Rojas

Carmen Rubio

Chapter 1

The Molecular Mechanisms of the Ketogenic Diet in Epilepsy

Moisés Rubio-Osornio[1]
Rudy Luna[2]
Tarsila Elizabeth Juárez-Zepeda[3]
Leticia Granados-Rojas[3,*]
and Carmen Rubio[2,†]

[1]Departamento de Neuroquímica, Instituto Nacional de Neurología y Neurocirugía, Manuel Velasco Suárez, Mexico City, Mexico
[2]Departamento de Neurofisiología, Instituto Nacional de Neurología y Neurocirugía, Manuel Velasco Suárez, Mexico City, Mexico
[3]Laboratorio de Neurociencias II, Instituto Nacional de Pediatría, Mexico City, Mexico

Abstract

In light of the fact that patients with epilepsy have responded well to alternative therapies, some treatments have been proposed for the control of epileptic seizures. One of these is the ketogenic diet. This diet regime is characterized by a lower carbohydrate intake compared to typical diets, resulting in a decrease in the energy used for the biochemical and genetic processes implicated in epileptic seizures. A variety of mechanisms can be included in this process. For instance, hyperpolarization mediated by adenosine triphosphate (ATP)-sensitive potassium channels (K_{ATP} channels) is a crucial mechanism in this diet.

Inhibition of Wnt pathway signaling and β-catenin translocation to the cell nucleus are related to potassium channels (K^+) that increase at

---

[*] Corresponding Author's Email:lgranados_2000@yahoo.com.mx.
[†] Corresponding Author's Email: macaru4@yahoo.com.mx.

In: The Ketogenic Diet Reexamined
Editors: Leticia Granados-Rojas and Carmen Rubio
ISBN: 979-8-89113-543-7
© 2024 Nova Science Publishers, Inc.

the extracellular level, preventing the release of calcium (Ca^{2+}). This process is followed by hyperpolarization induced by Wnt ligands, which causes Ca^{2+} to activate the K^+ current. After applying the ketogenic diet as therapy, there is suppressed oxidative stress and greater resistance to metabolic stress, raising the threshold for ATP release, neuroprotection, and reduced reactive oxygen species (ROS) formation. Furthermore, the ketogenic diet has been shown to benefit the gut microbiome and increase anti-inflammatory processes. However, there is currently limited investigation on the possible therapeutic benefits of dietary therapy in epilepsy along with the genetic processes involved. However, the potential genes associated with Wnt pathways and their regulation through K_{ATP} channels to achieve lower epileptic seizures at the molecular level are described throughout this chapter.

Keywords: ketogenic diet, molecular mechanisms, epilepsy

Acronyms

ADP	Adenosine diphosphate
AMPK	Adenosine monophosphate-activated protein kinase
ASIC	Acid-sensing channels
ATP	Adenosine triphosphate
Bad	Bcl-2 associated activator of cell death
BHB	β-hydroxybutyrate
Ca^{2+}	Calcium
CAT	Catalase
Fzd	Frizzled receptor
GABA	Gamma-aminobutyric acid
GABAA-Rs	Gamma-aminobutyric acid type A receptors
GSH	Glutathione
K^+	Potassium
K2P	Two-pore domain K+ channels
K_{ATP}	Adenosine triphosphate-sensitive potassium channels
KB	Ketone bodies
KD	Ketogenic diet
LDH	Lactate dehydrogenase
MCT	Monocarboxylic transporters
mPT	Mitochondria permeability transition
mtDNA	Mitochondrial DNA

Nrf2	Nuclear factor erythroid 2-related factor 2
PPAR	Peroxisome proliferator-activated receptor
PUFAs	Polyunsaturated fatty acids
Rheb	Ras homologous enriched in brain
ROS	Reactive oxygen species
TCF/LEF	T-cell factor lymphoid promoter-binding factor
TSC2	Tuberin protein
UCPs	Uncoupling proteins

Introduction

Since 1990, research involving the Ketogenic Diet (KD) in the treatment of drug-resistant epilepsy has gained a lot of traction. However, it was first used to treat refractory epilepsy in 1921 (Wilder, 1921). Freeman et al., (2007) and Ułamek-Kozioł et al., (2019) found that almost half of those treated with KD had seen a reduction in seizure frequency, with 10-15% experiencing no seizures at all.

KD lowers blood glucose levels and allows the brain to utilize ketone bodies (KB) as a source of energy to control numerous pathways. Thus, resulting in an anticonvulsant effect. The crucial underlying mechanism of KD is chronic ketosis. It decreases synaptic excitability and stabilizes synapses, increasing the energy reserve of the brain, associated with mitochondrial biogenesis and function (D'Andrea et al., 2019). However, some studies have not established a direct link between seizure thresholds and blood β-hydroxybutyrate (BHB). Therefore, implying that the anticonvulsant impact of KD is not dependent on specific KB, but rather that KD protects against the onset of seizures without decreasing the intensity of seizures (Raffo et al., 2008).

On the other hand, no specific epileptic disorders from which KD could benefit have been identified. However, its efficacy has been demonstrated in glucose transporter 1 deficiency syndrome, Angelman syndrome, and tuberous sclerosis complex. Its anti-inflammatory properties have been postulated as a potential therapy in autoimmune epilepsy and encephalitis (Husari & Cervenka, 2020). The deficiency in pyruvate dehydrogenase has been attributed to a positive response related to KD. However, due to the inability to metabolize KB, KD is not suitable for some patients with primary carnitine deficits and β-oxidation abnormalities (Schoeler et al., 2020). In short-term investigations, a small percentage of patients have experienced side effects such as gastrointestinal discomfort and elevated serum lipids, preventing them from following the diet as a treatment (Dutton & Escayg, 2008; Martin-McGill et al., 2018).

Multiple mechanisms of KD have been shown to contribute to the reduction of epileptic seizures, including neurotransmitter control, gut microbiota regulation, inhibition of apoptotic factors, inflammation, reduction of oxidative stress, and improvement of mitochondrial biogenesis. While there is evidence of enhanced energy metabolism genes in the brain, these mechanisms are not yet completely understood. In light of this, the various mechanisms that can reduce neuronal excitability will be discussed throughout this chapter.

Reactive Oxygen Species

Seizures and epileptogenesis induce mitochondria to generate reactive oxygen species (ROS), resulting in oxidative stress and malfunction of cellular macromolecules, affecting adenosine triphosphate (ATP) generation and mitochondrial DNA (mtDNA) stability. This is related to hippocampus excitotoxicity and apoptosis, which promotes neuronal excitability (Chuang et al., 2004; Waldbaum & Patel, 2010). KD inhibits ROS formation in mitochondria (Rowley & Patel, 2013). The accumulation of ROS promotes oxidative stress, which plays a role in the genesis and development of seizures. KB may offer acetyl-CoA to boost ATP generation, while also inhibiting ROS development and the mitochondrial permeability transition pore (mPTP). These processes can protect the cell from oxidative damage and prevent excessive discharge of calcium (Ca^{2+}). β-hydroxybutyric acid (BHB) and acetoacetate (AcAc) have also been shown to reduce hydrogen peroxide activity in the hippocampus by improving catalase (CAT) activity and decreasing nicotinamide adenine dinucleotide (NAD^+) oxidation, suggesting a positive effect on epileptic activity (Maalouf et al., 2007; Kim et al., 2010; Kim et al., 2015).

The antioxidant effects of BHB can be mediated by inhibiting class I histone deacetylases. It stimulates the acetylation of histones H3 lysine 9 and H3 lysine 14, as well as the transcription of the FOXO3A gene (a member of the FOXO subfamily of forkhead transcription factors), resulting in antioxidant enzymes that include manganese superoxide dismutase and CAT (Rogawski et al., 2016). Class I histone deacetylases are inhibited by BHA. BHB increases gene transcription on a large scale, especially in genes linked to resistance factors to oxidative stress. Increased acetyl-CoA promotes hyperacetylation of histones and non-histones, simultaneously blocking histone deacetylases and enhancing endogenous antioxidants (Shimazu et al., 2013; Simeone et al., 2018).

After a seizure, mitochondrial complex I and IV decrease, while an increase in complex II causes mitochondrial dysfunction due to oxidative stress, which is associated with a down-regulation in the encoded proteins for the electron transport chain. The above is crucial for membrane permeability, neurotransmitter biosynthesis, and ATP production, among other functions, resulting in an increase in ROS, which in the case of dysfunction leads to continuous oxidative stress. Due to the metabolism of fatty acids by the peroxisome proliferator activated receptor (PPAR) and the enhancement of FOX, KD could prevent the inhibition of mitochondrial complex I, II, and III and increase the number of uncoupling proteins (UCPs), decreasing oxidative stress in the brain and expressing antioxidant proteins that make the brain more resistant to oxidative stress (Yang et al., 2019).

ROS, on the other hand, promotes the transcription factor NF-E2-related factor 2 (Nrf2). It activates genes involved in antioxidant pathways, including those involved in the production and conjugation of reduced glutathione (GSH). In rats with temporal lobe epilepsy, Nrf2 expression reduces seizures (Mazzuferi et al., 2013). KD induces an endoplasmic buildup of Nrf2 in rats, and also enhances the activity of its target enzyme, nicotinamide adenine dinucleotide phosphate (NADPH): quinone oxidoreductase, in the hippocampus. ATP regulates transporters responsible for membrane potential and homeostasis, thereby improving synaptic transmission and increasing seizure resistance (Longo et al., 2019). Upon KD, increased mitochondrial function boosts GSH levels and production in the hippocampus, resulting in decreased levels of ROS such as hydrogen peroxide and improved mtDNA. After the KD treatment, there is an elevation of 4-hydroxy-2 nonenal, a lipid peroxidation product. This leads to the activation of a protective transcription factor pathway involving the Nrf2 protein, which promotes GSH biosynthesis through gene transcription (Milder et al., 2010).

After being suppressed by oxidative stress, mitochondrial permeability transition (mPT) is suggested to be the cause of cell death prevention due to KD treatment. KB work is similar to cyclosporine A, which raises the Ca^{2+} induced mPT opening threshold (Kim et al., 2007). It also lowers brain pH by blocking proton-sensitive ion channels and stimulating monocarboxylic transporters, proteins that transfer KB to the brain, such as MCT1 (Sook et al., 2004) (Figure 1).

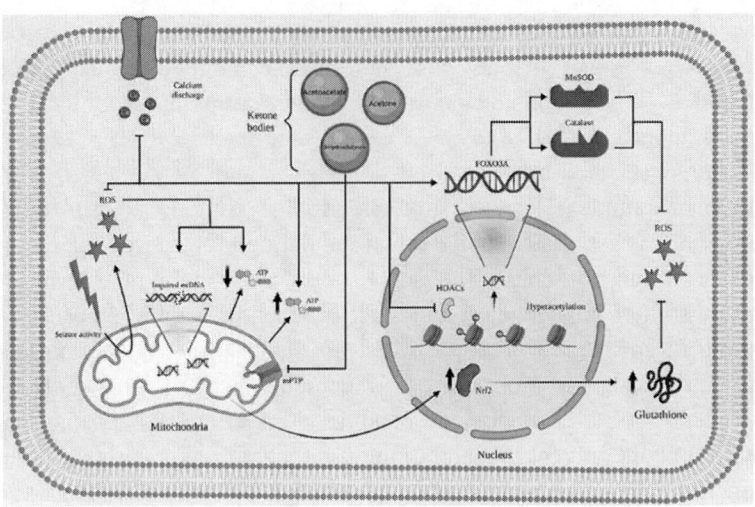

Figure 1. Reactive oxygen species (ROS). Cell discharge causes Ca2+ to enter the cytoplasm and promote seizure genesis. This leads mitochondria to generate ROS and induce oxidative stress and cellular malfunction that affect ATP generation. Ketone bodies boost ATP generation while protecting the cell from oxidative stress and inhibiting ROS formation in mitochondria by enhancing the function of FOXO3A, Nrf2, ATP: Adenosine triphosphate; Nrf2: Nuclear factor erythroid 2-related factor 2.

K_{ATP} Channels

Currently, ion channels are being studied as a possible explanation for the ketogenic effect of restrictive diets on the neuronal membrane potential. The KD activates the K_{ATP} channels, which improves mitochondrial metabolism and thus ATP generation. Due to their reactivity and sensitivity to changes in ATP concentrations, these channels are a part of the cell's metabolic status and membrane potential.

As a result, high concentrations of intracellular ATP inhibit the channels, whereas adenosine diphosphate (ADP) activates them, resulting in changes in the neuronal membrane potential by allowing changes in K^+ ion conductance, which hyperpolarize neurons and reduce neural excitability and epileptic seizures (DeVivo et al., 1978; Nakazawa et al., 1983; Nylen et al., 2009) (Figure 2).

K_{ATP} channels can be found in many different parts of the brain. Glucose-sensitive activities are highly expressed in this gene. In a resting state, K_{ATP} channels in the neuronal membrane are blocked, except in states of acute metabolic deprivation (anoxia and ischemia), which together cause cellular stress (Pierrefiche et al., 1996; Karschin et al., 1997; Dunn-Meynell et al., 1998; Zawar et al., 1999; Allen & Brown, 2004).

In excitatory neurons, KB hydrolyzes ATP through pannexin channels to produce adenosine, which activates inhibitory adenosine A1 receptors while also indirectly opening K_{ATP} channels, resulting in antiseizure effects, as demonstrated in experimental mice after lowering adenosine expression due to inhibition of adenosine kinase (Kawamura et al., 2010; Masino et al., 2011). The adenosine monophosphate-activated protein kinase (AMPK) enzyme is required for neural energy consumption during epileptic seizures. Inhibition of AMPK activity induces a reduction in K_{ATP} channels by phosphorylating two channel sites (s440 and s537), resulting in membrane hyperpolarization (Ikematsu et al., 2011).

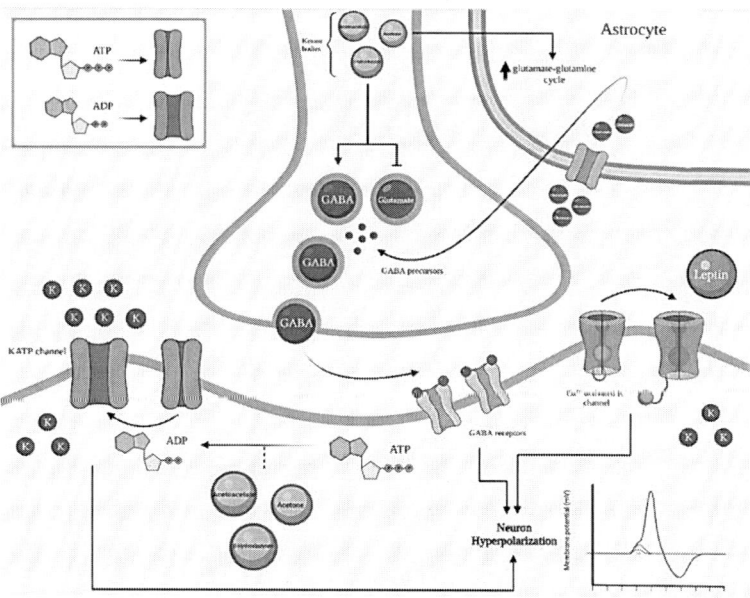

Figure 2. KATP channels. The KATP channels let K+ hyperpolarize neurons and reduce neural excitability. Ketone bodies produces adenosine by hydrolyzing ATP to ADP. This indirectly opens KATP channels, hyperpolarizing the neuron and inducing GABA formation and release. Thus, it promotes the antiseizure effect. KATP: Adenosine triphosphate-sensitive potassium channels; ATP: Adenosine triphosphate; ADP: Adenosine dipshosphate; GABA: Gamma-aminobutyric acid.

AMPK up-regulates the Bcl2 modifying factor gene, which prevents neuronal death in CA1 and CA3 of the hippocampus caused by seizures. It also encourages the Bcl-2-associated death-promotor (Bad) protein to reduce glucose metabolism in neurons while increasing metabolically sensitive K_{ATP} channel activity, resulting in in vivo seizure resistance to behavioral and electrographic seizures. Bad ablation reduces the activity of the hippocampal-entorhinal circuit in epileptiform neurons, protecting them against seizures produced by K_{ATP} channel activity (Giménez-Cassina et al., 2012; Yang et al., 2019; Martínez-François et al., 2018). Two-pore domain K^+ channels (K2P) are spontaneously active, resulting in a constant efflux of K^+ ions through the cell membrane, necessary to maintain the hyperpolarized resting potential of the cell membrane. These channels are thought to be activated by KB and certain fatty acids. The excitability of neuron membranes may be affected by K2P activation (Vamecq et al., 2005; Hughes et al., 2017; Barzegar et al., 2021).

Wnt Signaling Pathway

In experimental animals, higher Wnt/β-catenin signaling pathway is associated with a greater presence of seizures and even apoptosis (Rubio et al., 2017). The Wnt signaling pathway affects glucose regulatory mechanisms, causing cortical neurons to absorb more glucose. After generating a positive ion output, a reduction in glycolytic pathways combined with a rise in KB results in lower cytoplasmic ATP, which activates K_{ATP} channels and reduces cellular excitability (Ma et al., 2007). Wnt3a stimulation of cortical neurons increases glucose absorption without affecting the expression or functionality of glucose transporter 3 but does enhance its affinity. Furthermore, activation of the same ligand stimulates the activity of the two glycolysis regulating enzymes (hexokinase and 6-phosphorus-2-kinase/fructose-2,3-bisphosphatase) activity, directly related to glucose absorption as glucose increases (Cisternas et al., 2016). The AKT and Wnt pathways contribute to the increase in glucose by promoting glycogen synthesis in rapamycin proteins by inhibiting 3-kinase-glycogen synthase (Manning et al., 2002; Patel & Woodgett, 2017).

Mutations in genes involved in gluconeogenesis and glutamine metabolism in hepatocytes have also been found as a result of changes in the Wnt/β-catenin signaling pathways. Several of these involved proteins are related to mitochondrial dysfunction and carbohydrate metabolism, indicating that Wnt signaling abnormalities may lead to a metabolic shift in cell energy consumption away from fatty acid oxidation and toward glycolysis (Chafey et al., 2009). However, the significance of Wnt/β-catenin signaling pathways in glycolytic pathways, as well as their indirect role in epileptic neurons' cell membrane activity, is not yet fully understood. Because they regulate crucial processes such as hippocampus neurogenesis, synaptic cleft formation, and mitochondrial function, Wnt signaling pathways are critical for the development and functioning of the central nervous system (Budnik & Salinas, 2011; Inestrosa & Varela-Nallar, 2014).

The canonical pathway (β-catenin-dependent signaling pathway) and the non-canonical pathway (β-catenin-independent signaling pathway) are the two main pathways for Wnt signals. The former has been linked to the control of transcriptional activity and activation of genes such as c-Myc, cyclin D, and the T cell factor/lymphoid promoter-binding factor (TCF/LEF) pathway, which controls cell determination, cell proliferation, and stem cell differentiation.

Intracellular heterotrimeric activation of G proteins and disheveled proteins occurs when specific Wnt receptors (such as Wnt1, Wnt10b, or Wnt3a) bind to their Frizzled (Fzd)-LRP5 or Fzd-LRP6 receptors, which in the dentate gyrus leads to phosphorylation and recruitment of Axin to LRP5 (or LRP6) (Tamai et al., 2004; Nusse, 2005). By increasing its stabilization and accumulation in the cytoplasm, the aforementioned promotes the separation of β-catenin and the degradation complex. The above leads to the dissociation of β-catenin and the degradation complex by promoting its stabilization and accumulation of the molecule in the cytosol, therefore, it is translocated towards the nucleus and activates transcription factors of the TCF/LEF families, c-Myc and Cyclin D. Certain intracellular molecules expressed by Wnt-dependent activation of β-catenin jointly participate in the CA1 pyramidal cells of the region hippocampal and can increase sensitivity to pentylenetetrazole and kainate by inducing seizures and cell death (Koeller et al., 2008; Chien et al., 2009). Due to gene triggering, the open K_{ATP} channels release ROS, which increases mitochondrial synthesis. When K_{ATP} channels are blocked, Ca^{2+} is released into the nucleus, causing the c-Myc gene to be expressed (Quesada et al., 2002). However, in rats with repeated generalized seizures, the overexpression effect of β-catenin on c-Myc and cyclin D induces neuronal death in Purkinje cells and the cerebellum granule layer. Overexpression of c-Myc and cyclin D can be induced by activating β-catenin, which has an apoptotic effect by positively regulating and activating pro-apoptotic proteins (Rubio et al., 2017).

Cell mobility is mostly mediated by the second Wnt-dependent or noncanonical pathway (Logan & Nusse, 2004). This route increases neuronal excitability by altering intracellular Ca^{2+} triggered by Wnt5a while simultaneously decreasing K^+ currents in pyramidal neurons of CA1 (McQuate et al., 2017). When Fzd receptors are activated by their Wnt ligand, the enzyme GSK3 is inhibited, resulting in activation of tuberin protein (TSC2) (Inoki et al., 2006). TSC2 inhibits the homologous Ras protein enriched with brain proteins (Rheb), a mTORC1 activator, in the absence of these signals. Inactivation of Rheb by TSC2 causes mTORC1 inhibition, and inhibition of TSC2 causes mTORC1 activation indirectly (Inoki et al., 2002).

Neurotransmitters and Hormones

The synthesis of GABA (Gamma-aminobutyric acid) neurotransmitter is improved, whereas glutamate generation is reduced due to KD (Rogawski et al., 2016). Consumption of oxaloacetate in the tricarboxylic acid cycle lowers aspartate levels, which has an inhibitory effect on glutamate decarboxylase and facilitates glutamate conversion to glutamine in astrocytes (Yudkoff et al., 2001; D'Andrea et al., 2019). KB inhibits vesicular glutamate transporters and modulates GABA type A receptors (GABAA-Rs), which compete with chloride for allosteric activation of glutamate transporters. This reduces glutamate release and excitatory synaptic transmission (Juge et al., 2010; Simeone, 2018).

In the hippocampus, agmatine levels rise as a consequence of KD. It appears to be another inhibitory neurotransmitter that inhibits N-methyl-D-Aspartate, histamine, and adrenaline receptors in particular. It has been shown to have a synergistic effect with antiepileptic medications such as valproate, phenobarbital, and vigabatrin. In this sense, serotonin, dopamine and noradrenaline, neurotransmitters involved in neuronal excitability and seizures, levels are also affected by KD (Weinshenker, 2008; Dahlin et al., 2012; Calderón et al., 2017).

Furthermore, through neurohormones involved in energy homeostasis, KD decreases weight gain and increases leptin (Thio et al., 2006). Increased leptin levels may contribute to the anticonvulsant effects of KD. In addition to alterations in serum levels of insulin, ghrelin, and cortisol due to leptin receptors throughout the brain. Leptin can serve as an anticonvulsant and activate Ca^{2+} activated K^+ channels throughout the brain (Shanley et al., 2002).

Endogenous neuromodulators galanin and neuropeptide Y can suppress excessive neuronal excitability. Glucose, whose levels in the blood are lowered under KD, suppresses these orexigenic neuropeptides. A high-fat diet can also increase galanin expression (Weinshenker, 2008). After KD, serum changes of neurotransmitters and various hormones involved in metabolism occur, resulting in activation or inhibition of the ion channel. Most of them are associated with a reduction in neural excitability.

Insufficient synaptic inhibition and receptor alterations, such as low levels of GABAA-Rs in the molecular layer of the dentate gyrus, are among the pathologic mechanisms that cause neuronal excitability and seizures in epilepsy (O'Donnell-Luria et al., 2019). KB affect excitability, intracellular metabolic changes, and cell gene expression in several ways, both directly and indirectly. Furthermore, it has been established that KD boosts GABAA-Rs by enhancing inhibition in the dentate gyrus, a region linked to epileptic activity (Bough et al., 2003). 2-deoxy-D-glucose has been shown to give neuroprotective effects against seizures by inhibiting glycolysis. This inhibition may reduce the ATP/ADP ratio (Garriga-Canut et al., 2006).

Because aspartate is generated by glutamate when glucose is not available and acts as an excitatory amino acid released after depolarization, raising its levels in the intrasynaptic region, it is thought to play a crucial role in hippocampal epileptogenesis. KD increases blood levels of branched chain amino acids, particularly high levels of leucine in the brain, which prevent glutamate from being transaminated to aspartate (Yudkoff et al., 2001). The reduction of oxaloacetate, which is transformed to aspartate by a transamination event, is another mechanism that supports the role of KD in lowering aspartate (Yudkoff et al., 2005).

By some yet to be fully understood mechanism, ketosis causes the activation of glutamate decarboxylase, resulting in lower glutamate levels and higher levels of GABA. The KD response changes the glutamate-glutamine cycle by enhancing the astrocytic glutamine route, removing glutamate from synaptic clefts, and returning it as a GABA precursor to the presynaptic neuron. Another possible mechanism is that after KD, GABAergic function through GABA type B receptors enhances voltage-sensitive Ca^{2+} channel inhibition, causing greater stability between neurons in the hippocampus and control over transport proteins and the Na^+/K^+-ATPase pump, leading to ionic homeostasis for longer than expected. After KD therapy, there is greater resistance to metabolic stress, raising the threshold for ATP release (Nishimura et al., 2005; Bough et al., 2006).

Neuroprotection

Cell death is prevalent after chronic epileptic seizures, resulting in cognitive impairment (Shaafi et al., 2014). KD prevents apoptosis and neurotoxicity by inhibiting caspase 3 and increasing the amount of calbindin, which regulates intracellular Ca^{2+}. In neutrophils and macrophages, KB controls inflammation in response to PAMPs and DAMPs by activating HCA2 receptors and preventing activation of the NLRP3 inflammasome. Furthermore, interleukin 1b, HMGB1, and other pro-inflammatory cytokines are also reduced in the periphery and brain (Shimazu et al., 2013; Dupuis et al., 2015; Youm et al., 2015). The inflammatory response, which plays a critical role in the causation, severity, and neuronal death of seizures, is suppressed by KD via KB. In patients with refractory epilepsy, proinflammatory mediators could be a target for KD treatment.

Fatty Acids

By blocking voltage-gated sodium and Ca^{2+} channels, activating K2P channels, and improving $Na^+/K^+/ATPase$ pump activity, KD increases fatty acid oxidation by increasing the levels of polyunsaturated fatty acids (PUFAs) from adipose tissue to the liver and brain, which can reduce neuronal excitability and mitigate seizures (Michael-Titus and Priestley, 2014). PPAR is activated by PUFA, and regulates neurotransmitter metabolism and inhibits neuroinflammation. By reducing ROS generation, PUFAs also promote the expression of UCPs in mitochondria (Sullivan et al., 2004; Bough et al., 2007).

Gut Microbiome

Different forms of KD may have an impact on the diversity of the gut microbiota. Some studies show that pro-inflammatory bacteria have a favorable consequence on the architecture and function of bacteria in the gut; while others show that pro-inflammatory bacteria have a negative impact (Ellerbroek, 2018; Cabrera-Mulero et al., 2019). Antiseizure effects on the microbiome are suggested by the presence of bacteroidetes and proteobacteria, notably Akkermansia muciniphila and parabacteroides (Sourbron et al., 2020). Due to a reduction in carbohydrates, KD reduces Faecalibacterium, Blautia,

Bifidobacterium, and Eubacterium rectale bacteria, lowering fermentation, associated with an increase in GABA in the hypothalamus (Paoli et al., 2019; Lindefeldt et al., 2019).

By changing synaptic protein expression, long-term potentiation, and myelination, metabolites produced by these specific bacteria aid in inhibitory neurotransmitter production involved in seizures. The decrease in some peripheral gamma-glutamyl amino acids caused by KD is believed to lead to a higher amount of GABA in the hippocampus compared to glutamate. Antibiotics, such as metronidazole, ampicillin, penicillin, and other B-lactams, have been shown to cause seizures due to depletion of the microbiota (Sutter et al., 2015; Olson et al., 2018; Fan et al., 2019).

Acid-Sensing Channels

Acid-sensing channels (ASIC) are inhibited by the KB. ASIC has a modulatory influence on GABAergic transmission in the GABAergic synapses of the hippocampus, crucial in its neuroprotective activity. Due to anaerobic metabolism that results in brain injury, these channels are active during epileptic seizures, ischemia, and poisoning (Storozhuk et al., 2016; Zhu et al., 2019).

Lactate Dehydrogenase

LDHA, a subunit of lactate dehydrogenase (LDH), is part of the lactic interaction between the neuron and the astrocyte. In contrast to the LDHB subunit, it has a hyperpolarizing effect on the neuron in persistent seizures. This is the first prospective antiepileptic drug that mimics the action of the KD anticonvulsant that can target the LDH pathway (Sada et al., 2015; Sada et al., 2020).

Conclusion

The goal has been to define the various action mechanisms in order to better understand how this alternative antiepileptic treatment could aid seizure management. KD has been shown to reduce seizures by producing KB, which influences neuronal activity and neurotransmitter release, such as reduced glutamate, improved mitochondrial function, increased GABA synthesis, and activation of K_{ATP} channels. There appears to be a relationship between all of the anticonvulsant effects of KD leading to alterations of AMPK and ATP and up-regulation/down-regulation of the protein, implying that the electron transport chain in the mitochondria is improved and, as a result, energy sources are better utilized. KD, on the other hand, has the potential to impede glycolysis. It helps in mitochondrial biogenesis, oxidative stress reduction, and inflammation reduction. The electrophysiological response to epileptic seizures is modulated by molecular alterations that intervene in the glycolytic metabolism of neurons.

Identifying the metabolic pathways that interfere with the operation of K_{ATP} channels in neurons with epileptiform crises is critical because evidence proposes that they could be used as a potential pharmacological target for new generation of treatment aimed to transform these metabolic processes. Despite this, there is insufficient evidence to suggest a specific treatment related to these genes and their association with K_{ATP} channels to manage epileptic seizures due to a lack of research and small sample sizes.

References

Allen, T. G. J., & Brown, D. A. (2004). Modulation of the excitability of cholinergic basal forebrain neurons by K_{ATP} channels. *The Journal of Physiology, 554*(2), 353–370. doi: 10.1113/jphysiol.2003.055889.

Barzegar, M., Afghan, M., Tarmahi, V., Behtari, M., Rahimi Khamaneh, S., & Raeisi, S. (2021). Ketogenic diet: Overview, types, and possible anti-seizure mechanisms. *Nutritional Neuroscience, 24*(4), 307–316. doi: 10.1080/1028415X.2019.1627769.

Bough, K. J., Schwartzkroin, P. A., & Rho, J. M. (2003). Calorie restriction and ketogenic diet diminish neuronal excitability in rat dentate gyrus in vivo. *Epilepsia, 44*(6), 752–760. doi: 10.1046/j.1528-1157.2003.55502.x.

Bough, K. J., Wetherington, J., Hassel, B., Pare, J. F., Gawryluk, J. W., Greene, J. G., Shaw, R., Smith, Y., Geiger, J. D., & Dingledine, R. J. (2006). Mitochondrial biogenesis in the anticonvulsant mechanism of the ketogenic diet. *Annals of Neurology, 60*(2), 223–235. doi: 10.1002/ana.20899.

Bough, K. J., & Rho, J. M. (2007). Anticonvulsant mechanisms of the ketogenic diet. *Epilepsia, 48*(1), 43–58. doi: 10.1111/j.1528-1167.2007.00915.x.

Budnik, V., & Salinas, P. C. (2011). Wnt signaling during synaptic development and plasticity. *Current Opinion in Neurobiology, 21*(1), 151–159. doi: 1016/j.conb.2010.12.002.

Cabrera-Mulero, A., Tinahones, A., Bandera, B., Moreno-Indias, I., Macías-González, M., & Tinahones, F. J. (2019). Keto microbiota: A powerful contributor to host disease recovery. *Reviews in Endocrine and Metabolic Disorders, 20*(4), 415–425. doi: 1007/s11154-019-09518-8.

Calderón, N., Betancourt, L., Hernández, L., & Rada, P. (2017). A ketogenic diet modifies glutamate, gamma-aminobutyric acid and agmatine levels in the hippocampus of rats: A microdialysis study. *Neuroscience Letters,* 6, 158–162. doi: 10.1016/j.neulet.2017.02.014.

Chafey, P., Finzi, L., Boisgard, R., Caüzac, M., Clary, G., Broussard, C., Pégorier, J. P., Guillonneau, F., Mayeux, P., Camoin, L., Tavitian, B., Colnot, S., & Perret, C. (2009). Proteomic analysis of β-catenin activation in mouse liver by DIGE analysis identifies glucose metabolism as a new target of the Wnt pathway. *Proteomics, 9*(14), 3889-3900. doi: 10.1002/pmic.200800609.

Chien, A. J., Conrad, W. H., & Moon, R. T. (2009). A Wnt survival guide: From flies to human disease. *Journal of Investigative Dermatology, 129*(7), 1614–1627. doi: 10.1038/jid.2008.445.

Chuang, Y. C., Chang, A. Y. W., Lin, J. W., Hsu, S. P., & Chan, S. H. H. (2004). Mitochondrial dysfunction and ultrastructural damage in the hippocampus during kainic acid-induced status epilepticus in the rat. *Epilepsia*, 45(9), 1202–1209. doi: 1111/j.0013-9580.2004.18204.x.

Cisternas, P., Salazar, P., Silva-Álvarez, C., Barros, L. F., & Inestrosa, N. C. (2016). Activation of Wnt signaling in cortical neurons enhances glucose utilization through glycolysis. *Journal of Biological Chemistry, 291*(50), 25950–25964. doi: 10.1074/jbc.M116.735373.

Dahlin, M., Månsson, J. E., & Åmark, P. (2012). CSF levels of dopamine and serotonin, but not norepinephrine, metabolites are influenced by the ketogenic diet in children with epilepsy. *Epilepsy Research, 99*(1–2), 132–138. doi: 10.1016/j.eplepsyres.2011.11.003.

D'Andrea, M. I., Romão, T. T., Pires do Prado, H. J., Krüger, L. T., Pires, M. E. P., & da Conceição, P. O. (2019). Ketogenic diet and epilepsy: What we know so far. *Frontiers in Neuroscience, 13*, 5. doi: 10.3389/fnins.2019.00005.

DeVivo, D. C., Leckie, M. P., Ferrendelli, J. S., & McDougal, D. B. (1978). Chronic ketosis and cerebral metabolism. *Annals of Neurology, 3*(4), 331–337. doi: 1002/ana.410030410.

Dunn-Meynell, A. A., Rawson, N. E., & Levin, B. E. (1998). Distribution and phenotype of neurons containing the ATP-sensitive K^+ channel in rat brain. *Brain Research, 814*(1–2), 41–54. doi: 10.1016/S0006-8993(98)00956-1.

Dupuis, N., Curatolo, N., Benoist, J. F., & Auvin, S. (2015). Ketogenic diet exhibits anti-inflammatory properties. *Epilepsia, 56*(7), e95–e98. doi: 10.1111/epi.13038.

Dutton, S. B. B., & Escayg, A. (2008). Genetic influences on ketogenic diet efficacy. *Epilepsia, 49*(Suppl. 8), 67–69. doi: 10.1111/j.1528-1167.2008.01839.x.

Ellerbroek, A. (2018). The effect of ketogenic diets on the gut microbiota. *Journal of Exercise and Nutrition, 1*(5). https://www.journalofexerciseandnutrition.com/index.php/JEN/article/view/32.

Fan, Y., Wang, H., Liu, X., Zhang, J., & Liu, G. (2019). Crosstalk between the ketogenic diet and epilepsy: From the perspective of gut microbiota. *Mediators of Inflammation, 2019*, 8373060. doi: 10.1155/2019/8373060.

Freeman, J. M., Kossoff, E. H., & Hartman, A. L. (2007). The ketogenic diet: One decade later. *Pediatrics, 119*(3), 535–543. doi: 10.1542/peds.2006-2447.

Garriga-Canut, M., Schoenike, B., Qazi, R., Bergendahl, K., Daley, T. J., Pfender, R. M., Morrison, J. F., Ockuly, J., Stafstrom, C., Sutula, T., & Roopra, A. (2006). 2-Deoxy-D-glucose reduces epilepsy progression by NRSF-CtBP–dependent metabolic regulation of chromatin structure. *Nature Neuroscience, 9*(11), 1382–1387. doi: 10.1038/nn1791.

Giménez-Cassina, A., Martínez-François, J. R., Fisher, J. K., Szlyk, B., Polak, K., Wiwczar, J., Tanner, G. R., Lutas, A., Yellen, G., & Danial, N. N. (2012). BAD-Dependent regulation of fuel metabolism and K_{ATP} channel activity confers resistance to epileptic seizures. *Neuron, 74*(4), 719–730. doi: 10.1016/j.neuron.2012.03.032.

Hughes, S., Foster, R. G., Peirson, S. N., & Hankins, M. W. (2017). Expression and localisation of two-pore domain (K2P) background leak potassium ion channels in the mouse retina. *Scientific Reports, 7*, 46085. doi: 10.1038/srep46085.

Husari, K. S., & Cervenka, M. C. (2020). The ketogenic diet all grown up–ketogenic diet therapies for adults. *Epilepsy Research, 162*, 106319. doi: 10.1016/j.eplepsyres.2020.106319.

Ikematsu, N., Dallas, M. L., Ross, F. A., Lewis, R. W., Rafferty, J. N., David, J. A., Suman, R., Peers, C., Hardie, D. G., & Evans, A. M. (2011). Phosphorylation of the voltage-gated potassium channel Kv2.1 by AMP-activated protein kinase regulates membrane excitability. *Proceedings of the National Academy of Sciences of United States of America, 108*(44), 18132–18137. doi: 10.1073/pnas.1106201108.

Inestrosa, N. C., & Varela-Nallar, L. (2014). Wnt signaling in the nervous system and in Alzheimer's disease. *Journal of Molecular Cell Biology, 6*(1), 64–74. doi: 10.1093/jmcb/mjt051.

Inoki, K., Li, Y., Zhu, T., Wu, J., & Guan, K. L. (2002). TSC2 is phosphorylated and inhibited by Akt and suppresses mTOR signalling. *Nature Cell Biology, 4*(9), 648–657. doi: 10.1038/ncb839.

Inoki, K., Ouyang, H., Zhu, T., Lindvall, C., Wang, Y., Zhang, X., Yang, Q., Bennett, C., Harada, Y., Stankunas, K., Wang, C., He, X., MacDougald, O. A., You, M., Williams, B. O., & Guan, K. L. (2006). TSC2 integrates Wnt and energy signals via a coordinated phosphorylation by AMPK and GSK3 to regulate cell growth. *Cell, 126*(5), 955–968. doi: 10.1016/j.cell.2006.06.055.

Juge, N., Gray, J. A., Omote, H., Miyaji, T., Inoue, T., Hara, C., Uneyama, H., Edwards, R. H., Nicoll, R. A., & Moriyama, Y. (2010). Metabolic control of vesicular glutamate transport and release. *Neuron, 68*(1), 99–112. doi: 10.1016/j.neuron.2010.09.002.

Karschin, C., Ecke, C., Ashcroft, F. M., & Karschin, A. (1997). Overlapping distribution of K_{ATP} channel-forming Kir6.2 subunit and the sulfonylurea receptor SUR1 in rodent brain. *FEBS Letters, 401*(1), 59–64. doi: 10.1016/S0014-5793(96)01438-X.

Kawamura, M., Ruskin, D. N., & Masino, S. A. (2010). Metabolic autocrine regulation of neurons involves cooperation among pannexin hemichannels, adenosine receptors, and K$_{ATP}$ channels. *Journal of Neuroscience, 30*(11), 3886–3895. doi: 10.1523/JNEUROSCI.0055-10.2010.

Kim, D. Y., Davis, L. M., Sullivan, P. G., Maalouf, M., Simeone, T. A., Brederode, J., & Rho, J. M. (2007). Ketone bodies are protective against oxidative stress in neocortical neurons. *Journal of Neurochemistry, 101*(5), 1316–1326. doi: 10.1111/j.1471-4159.2007.04483.x.

Kim, D. Y., Vallejo, J., & Rho, J. M. (2010). Ketones prevent synaptic dysfunction induced by mitochondrial respiratory complex inhibitors. *Journal of Neurochemistry, 114*(1), 130–141. doi: 10.1111/j.1471-4159.2010.06728.x.

Kim, D. Y., Simeone, K. A., Simeone, T. A., Pandya, J. D., Wilke, J. C., Ahn, Y., Geddes, J. W., Sullivan, P. G., & Rho, J. M. (2015). Ketone bodies mediate antiseizure effects through mitochondrial permeability transition. *Annals of Neurology, 78*(1), 77–87. doi: 10.1002/ana.24424.

Koeller, H. B., Ross, M. E., & Glickstein, S. B. (2008). Cyclin D1 in excitatory neurons of the adult brain enhances kainate-induced neurotoxicity. *Neurobiology of Disease, 31*(2), 230–241. doi: 10.1016/j.nbd.2008.04.010.

Lindefeldt, M., Eng, A., Darban, H., Bjerkner, A., Zetterström, C. K., Allander, T., Andersson, B., Borenstein, E., Dahlin, M., & Prast-Nielsen, S. (2019). The ketogenic diet influences taxonomic and functional composition of the gut microbiota in children with severe epilepsy. *Npj Biofilms and Microbiomes, 5*(5), 2–13 doi: 10.1038/s41522-018-0073-2.

Logan, C. Y., & Nusse, R. (2004). The Wnt signaling pathway in development and disease. *Annual Review of Cell and Developmental Biology, 20*, 781–810. doi: 10.1146/annurev.cellbio.20.010403.113126.

Longo, R., Peri, C., Cricrì, D., Coppi, L., Caruso, D., Mitro, N., de Fabiani, E., & Crestani, M. (2019). Ketogenic diet: A new light shining on old but gold biochemistry. *Nutrients, 11*(10), 2497. doi: 10.3390/nu11102497.

Ma, W., Berg, J., & Yellen, G. (2007). Ketogenic diet metabolites reduce firing in central neurons by opening K$_{ATP}$ channels. *Journal of Neuroscience, 27*(14), 3618–3625. doi: 10.1523/JNEUROSCI.0132-07.2007.

Maalouf, M., Sullivan, P. G., Davis, L., Kim, D. Y., & Rho, J. M. (2007). Ketones inhibit mitochondrial production of reactive oxygen species production following glutamate excitotoxicity by increasing NADH oxidation. *Neuroscience, 145*(1), 256–264. doi: 10.1016/j.neuroscience.2006.11.065.

Manning, B. D., Tee, A. R., Logsdon, M. N., Blenis, J., & Cantley, L. C. (2002). Identification of the tuberous sclerosis complex-2 tumor suppressor gene product tuberin as a target of the phosphoinositide 3-Kinase/Akt pathway. *Molecular Cell, 10*(1), 151–162. doi: 10.1016/S1097-2765(02)00568-3.

Martínez-François, J. R., Fernández-Agüera, M. C., Nathwani, N., Lahmann, C., Burnham, V. L., Danial, N. N., & Yellen, G. (2018). BAD and K$_{ATP}$ channels regulate neuron excitability and epileptiform activity. *ELife, 7*, e32721. doi: 10.7554/eLife.32721.

Martin-McGill, K. J., Jackson, C. F., Bresnahan, R., Levy, R. G., & Cooper, P. N. (2018). Ketogenic diets for drug-resistant epilepsy. *Cochrane Database of Systematic Reviews, 11*, 001903. doi: 10.1002/14651858.CD001903.pub4.

Masino, S. A., Li, T., Theofilas, P., Sandau, U. S., Ruskin, D. N., Fredholm, B. B., Geiger, J. D., Aronica, E., & Boison, D. (2011). A ketogenic diet suppresses seizures in mice through adenosine A1 receptors. *Journal of Clinical Investigation, 121*(7), 2679-2683. doi: 10.1172/JCI57813.

Mazzuferi, M., Kumar, G., Van Eyll, J., Danis, B., Foerch, P., & Kaminski, R. M. (2013). Nrf2 defense pathway: Experimental evidence for its protective role in epilepsy. *Annals of Neurology, 74*(4), 560–568. doi: 10.1002/ana.23940.

McQuate, A., Latorre-Esteves, E., & Barria, A. (2017). A Wnt/Calcium signaling cascade regulates neuronal excitability and trafficking of NMDARs. *Cell Reports, 21*(1), 60–69. doi: 10.1016/j.celrep.2017.09.023.

Michael-Titus, A. T., & Priestley, J. V. (2014). Omega-3 fatty acids and traumatic neurological injury: from neuroprotection to neuroplasticity? *Trends in Neurosciences, 37*(1), 30–38. doi: 10.1016/j.tins.2013.10.005.

Milder, J. B., Liang, L. P., & Patel, M. (2010). Acute oxidative stress and systemic Nrf2 activation by the ketogenic diet. *Neurobiology of Disease, 40*(1), 238–244. doi: 10.1016/j.nbd.2010.05.030.

Nakazawa, M., Kodama, S., & Matsuo, T. (1983). Effects of ketogenic diet on electroconvulsive threshold and brain contents of adenosine nucleotides. *Brain and Development, 5*(4), 375–380. doi: 10.1016/S0387-7604(83)80042-4.

Nishimura, T., Schwarzer, C., Gasser, E., Kato, N., Vezzani, A., & Sperk, G. (2005). Altered expression of GABAa and GABAb receptor subunit mRNAs in the hippocampus after kindling and electrically induced status epilepticus. *Neuroscience, 134*(2), 691–704. doi: 10.1016/j.neuroscience.2005.04.013.

Nusse, R. (2005). Relays at the membrane. *Nature, 438*, 747–749. doi: 10.1038/438747a.

Nylen, K., Velazquez, J. L. P., Sayed, V., Gibson, K. M., Burnham, W. M., & Snead, O. C. (2009). The effects of a ketogenic diet on ATP concentrations and the number of hippocampal mitochondria in Aldh5a1−/− mice. *Biochimica et Biophysica Acta, 1790*(3), 208–212. doi: 10.1016/j.bbagen.2008.12.005.

O'Donnell-Luria, A. H., Pais, L. S., Faundes, V., Wood, J. C., Sveden, A., Luria, V., Abou Jamra, R., Accogli, A., Amburgey, K., Anderlid, B. M., Azzarello-Burri, S., Basinger, A. A., Bianchini, C., Bird, L. M., Buchert, R., Carre, W., Ceulemans, S., Charles, P., Cox, H., & Hurles, M. E. (2019). Heterozygous variants in KMT2E cause a spectrum of neurodevelopmental disorders and epilepsy. *The American Journal of Human Genetics, 104*(6), 1210–1222. doi: 10.1016/j.ajhg.2019.03.021.

Olson, C. A., Vuong, H. E., Yano, J. M., Liang, Q. Y., Nusbaum, D. J., & Hsiao, E. Y. (2018). The gut microbiota mediates the anti-seizure effects of the ketogenic diet. *Cell, 173*(7), 1728–1741.e13. doi: 10.1016/j.cell.2018.04.027.

Paoli, A., Mancin, L., Bianco, A., Thomas, E., Mota, J. F., & Piccini, F. (2019). Ketogenic diet and microbiota: Friends or enemies? *Genes, 10*, 534. doi: 10.3390/genes10070534.

Patel, P., & Woodgett, J. R. (2017). Glycogen synthase kinase 3: A kinase for all pathways. *Current Topics in Developmental Biology, 123*, 277–302. doi: 10.1016/bs.ctdb.2016.11.011.

Pierrefiche, O., Bischoff, A. M., & Richter, D. W. (1996). ATP-sensitive K⁺ channels are functional in expiratory neurones of normoxic cats. *The Journal of Physiology, 494*(2), 399-409. doi: 10.1113/jphysiol.1996.sp021501.

Quesada, I., Rovira, J. M., Martin, F., Roche, E., Nadal, A., & Soria, B. (2002). Nuclear K$_{ATP}$ channels trigger nuclear Ca^{2+} transients that modulate nuclear function. *Proceedings of the National Academy of Sciences of United State of America, 99*(14), 9544-9549. doi: 10.1073/pnas.142039299.

Raffo, E., François, J., Ferrandon, A., Koning, E., & Nehlig, A. (2008). Calorie-restricted ketogenic diet increases thresholds to all patterns of pentylenetetrazol-induced seizures: Critical importance of electroclinical assessment. *Epilepsia, 49*(2), 320-328. doi: 10.1111/j.1528-1167.2007.01380.x.

Rogawski, M. A., Löscher, W., & Rho, J. M. (2016). Mechanisms of action of antiseizure drugs and the ketogenic diet. *Cold Spring Harbor Perspectives in Medicine, 6*(5), a022780. doi: 10.1101/cshperspect.a022780.

Rowley, S., & Patel, M. (2013). Mitochondrial involvement and oxidative stress in temporal lobe epilepsy. *Free Radical Biology and Medicine, 62*, 121-131. doi: 10.1016/j.freeradbiomed.2013.02.002.

Rubio, C., Rosiles-Abonce, A., Trejo-Solis, C., Rubio-Osornio, M., Mendoza, C., Custodio, V., Martinez-Lazcano, J. C., Gonzalez, E., & Paz, C. (2017). Increase signaling of Wnt/β-Catenin pathway and presence of apoptosis in cerebellum of kindled rats. *CNS & Neurological Disorders, 16*(7), 772-780. doi: 10.2174/1871527316666170117114513.

Sada, N., Lee, S., Katsu, T., Otsuki, T., & Inoue, T. (2015). Targeting LDH enzymes with a stiripentol analog to treat epilepsy. *Science, 347*(6228), 126-133. doi: 10.1126/science.aaa1299.

Sada, N., Suto, S., Suzuki, M., Usui, S., & Inoue, T. (2020). Upregulation of lactate dehydrogenase A in a chronic model of temporal lobe epilepsy. *Epilepsia, 61*(5), e37-e42. doi: 10.1111/epi.16488.

Schoeler, N. E., Simpson, Z., Whiteley, V. J., Nguyen, P., Meskell, R., Lightfoot, K., Martin-McGill, K. J., Olpin, S., & Ivison, F. (2020). Biochemical assessment of patients following ketogenic diets for epilepsy: Current practice in the UK and Ireland. *Epilepsia Open, 5*(1), 73-79. doi: 10.1002/epi4.12371.

Shaafi, S., Mahmoudi, J., Pashapour, A., Farhoudi, M., Sadigh-Eteghad, S., & Akbari, H. (2014). Ketogenic diet provides neuroprotective effects against ischemic stroke neuronal damages. *Advanced Pharmaceutical Bulletin, 4*(Suppl 2), 479-481. doi: 10.5681/apb.2014.071.

Shanley, L. J., Irving, A. J., Rae, M. G., Ashford, M. L. J., & Harvey, J. (2002). Leptin inhibits rat hippocampal neurons via activation of large conductance calcium-activated K⁺ channels. *Nature Neuroscience, 5*(4), 299-300. doi: 10.1038/nn824.

Shimazu, T., Hirschey, M. D., Newman, J., He, W., Shirakawa, K., le Moan, N., Grueter, C. A., Lim, H., Saunders, L. R., Stevens, R. D., Newgard, C. B., Farese, R. V., de Cabo, R., Ulrich, S., Akassoglou, K., & Verdin, E. (2013). Suppression of oxidative stress by β-hydroxybutyrate, an endogenous histone deacetylase inhibitor. *Science, 339*(6116), 211-214. doi: 10.1126/science.1227166.

Simeone, T. A., Simeone, K. A., Stafstrom, C. E., & Rho, J. M. (2018). Do ketone bodies mediate the anti-seizure effects of the ketogenic diet. *Neuropharmacology, 133*, 233–241. doi: 10.1016/j.neuropharm.2018.01.011.

Sook Noh, H., Po Lee, H., Wook Kim, D., Soo Kang, S., Jae Cho, G., Rho, J. M., & Sung Choi, W. (2004). A cDNA microarray analysis of gene expression profiles in rat hippocampus following a ketogenic diet. *Molecular Brain Research, 129*(1–2), 80–87. doi: 10.1016/j.molbrainres.2004.06.020.

Sourbron, J., Klinkenberg, S., Van Kuijk, S. M. J., Lagae, L., Lambrechts, D., Braakman, H. M. H., & Majoie, M. (2020). Ketogenic diet for the treatment of pediatric epilepsy: Review and meta-analysis. *Child's Nervous System, 36*(6), 1099–1109. doi: 10.1007/s00381-020-04578-7.

Storozhuk, M., Kondratskaya, E., Nikolaenko, L., & Krishtal, O. (2016). A modulatory role of ASICs on GABAergic synapses in rat hippocampal cell cultures. *Molecular Brain, 9*, 1–12. doi: 10.1186/s13041-016-0269-4.

Sullivan, P. G., Rippy, N. A., Dorenbos, K., Concepcion, R. C., Agarwal, A. K., & Rho, J. M. (2004). The ketogenic diet increases mitochondrial uncoupling protein levels and activity. *Annals of Neurology, 55*(4), 576–580. doi: 10.1002/ana.20062.

Sutter, R., Rüegg, S., & Tschudin-Sutter, S. (2015). Seizures as adverse events of antibiotic drugs. *Neurology, 85*(15), 1332–1341. doi: 10.1212/WNL.0000000000002023.

Tamai, K., Zeng, X., Liu, C., Zhang, X., Harada, Y., Chang, Z., & He, X. (2004). A mechanism for Wnt coreceptor activation. *Molecular Cell, 13*(1), 149–156. doi: 10.1016/S1097-2765(03)00484-2.

Thio, L. L., Erbayat-Altay, E., Rensing, N., & Yamada, K. A. (2006). Leptin contributes to slower weight gain in juvenile rodents on a ketogenic diet. *Pediatric Research, 60*(4), 413–417. doi: 10.1203/01.pdr.0000238244.54610.27.

Ułamek-Kozioł, M., Czuczwar, S. J., Januszewski, S., & Pluta, R. (2019). Ketogenic diet and epilepsy. *Nutrients, 11*(10), 2510. doi: 10.3390/nu11102510.

Vamecq, J., Vallee, L., Lesage, F., Gressens, P., & Stables, J. (2005). Antiepileptic popular ketogenic diet: emerging twists in an ancient story. *Progress in Neurobiology, 75*(1), 1–28. doi: 10.1016/j.pneurobio.2004.11.003.

Waldbaum, S., & Patel, M. (2010). Mitochondria, oxidative stress, and temporal lobe epilepsy. *Epilepsy Research, 88*(1), 23–45. doi: 10.1016/j.eplepsyres.2009.09.020.

Weinshenker, D. (2008). The contribution of norepinephrine and orexigenic neuropeptides to the anticonvulsant effect of the ketogenic diet. *Epilepsia, 49*(s8), 104–107. doi: 10.1111/j.1528-1167.2008.01850.x.

Wilder, R. M. (1921). The effects of ketonemia on the course of epilepsy. *Mayo Clinic Proceedings, 2*, 307–308.

Yang, H., Shan, W., Zhu, F., Wu, J., & Wang, Q. (2019). Ketone bodies in neurological diseases: Focus on neuroprotection and underlying mechanisms. *Frontiers in Neurology, 10*, 585. doi: 10.3389/fneur.2019.00585.

Youm, Y. H., Nguyen, K. Y., Grant, R. W., Goldberg, E. L., Bodogai, M., Kim, D., D'Agostino, D., Planavsky, N., Lupfer, C., Kanneganti, T. D., Kang, S., Horvath, T. L., Fahmy, T. M., Crawford, P. A., Biragyn, A., Alnemri, E., & Dixit, V. D. (2015). The ketone metabolite β-hydroxybutyrate blocks NLRP3 inflammasome–mediated inflammatory disease. *Nature Medicine, 21*(3), 263–269. doi: 10.1038/nm.3804.

Yudkoff, M., Daikhin, Y., Nissim, I., Lazarow, A., & Nissim, I. (2001). Ketogenic diet, amino acid metabolism, and seizure control. *Journal of Neuroscience Research, 66*(5), 931–940. doi: 10.1002/jnr.10083.

Yudkoff, M., Daikhin, Y., Nissim, I., Horyn, O., Lazarow, A., Luhovyy, B., Wehrli, S., & Nissim, I. (2005). Response of brain amino acid metabolism to ketosis. *Neurochemistry International, 47*(1–2), 119–128. doi: 10.1016/j.neuint.2005.04.014.

Zawar, C., Plant, T. D., Schirra, C., Konnerth, A., & Neumcke, B. (1999). Cell-type specific expression of ATP-sensitive potassium channels in the rat hippocampus. *The Journal of Physiology, 514*(2), 327–341. doi: 10.1111/j.1469-7793.1999.315ae.x.

Zhu, F., Shan, W., Xu, Q., Guo, A., Wu, J., & Wang, Q. (2019). Ketone bodies inhibit the opening of acid-sensing ion channels (ASICs) in rat hippocampal excitatory neurons in vitro. *Frontiers in Neurology, 10*, 155. doi: 10.3389/fneur.2019.00155.

Chapter 2

The Role of the Ketogenic Diet on Parkinson's Disease Symptoms

Joyce Graciela Martínez-Galindo[1]
Ana Vigil-Martínez[2]
and Ernesto Ochoa[3],*

[1]Laboratorio de Demencias, Instituto Nacional de Neurología y Neurocirugía, Manuel Velasco Suárez, Mexico City, Mexico
[2]Departamento de Fisiología de la Nutrición, Instituto Nacional de Ciencias Médicas y Nutrición, Salvador Zubirán, Mexico City, Mexico
[3]Departamento de Neurofisiología, Instituto Nacional de Neurología y Neurocirugía, Manuel Velasco Suárez, Mexico City, Mexico

Abstract

The ketogenic diet (KD) is a low-carbohydrate and fat-rich diet. It is implemented in the treatment of neurodegenerative disorders, including Parkinson's disease (PD), as recently explored. Although there is not much evidence, some studies in human patients and animal models of PD have shown a decrease in motor and non-motor symptoms of PD. The underlying mechanisms of the beneficial effects of KD on PD are not entirely understood. It is suggested that KD exerts neuroprotective and antioxidant effects. Thus, it leads to improved mitochondrial function and decreased neuroinflammation and oxidative stress, the primary pathogenetic triggers of the disease.

Keywords: ketogenic diet, Parkinson's disease, Parkinson's disease symptoms

In: The Ketogenic Diet Reexamined
Editors: Leticia Granados-Rojas and Carmen Rubio
ISBN: 979-8-89113-543-7
© 2024 Nova Science Publishers, Inc.

Acronyms

6-OHDA	6-Hydroxidopamine
AcAc	Acetoacetate
βHB	β-hydroxybutyrate
CKD	Classic ketogenic diet
CNS	Central nervous system
GLOBOCAN	Global Cancer Observatory
Gpe	External globus pallidus
GPi	Internal globus pallidus
GPx	Glutathione peroxidase
GSH	Glutathione
HMG-CoA	Hydroxymethylglutaril-CoA
KB	Ketone bodies
KD	Ketogenic diet
LCT	Long chain triglycerides
LGIT	Low glycemic index treatment
MAD	Modified Atkins diet
MCTD	Medium-chain triglyceride diet
NADH	Nicotinamide adenine dinucleotide
OS	Oxidative stress
PD	Parkinson disease
ROS	Reactive oxygen species
SNpr	Substantia nigra pars reticulata
STN	Subthalamic nucleus
UPDRS	Unified Parkinson's Disease Raiting Scale Unified
VA	Ventroanterior
VL	Ventrolateral

Introduction

The Ketogenic Diet (DK) is characterized by a high lipid, moderate protein and low carbohydrate content, including a state of ketosis, which simulates the metabolic effects observed in prolonged fasting. KD has been used as a therapeutic approach for some pathologies, particularly epilepsy (Zhu et al., 2022). Growing evidence suggests that KD could effectively improve symptoms in neurological disorders, including Parkinson's disease (PD) (Paoli et al., 2014; Pavón et al., 2021). According to the Parkinson Foundation (2022), PD is a neurodegenerative disorder that affects predominantly dopaminergic neurons in the *substantia nigra*. It is the second most common neurodegenerative disease. More than 10 million people worldwide are currently living with the disorder. The incidence increases with age, but an estimated 4% of people with PD are diagnosed before age 50, and men are 1.5 times more prone to the disorder (Bloem et al., 2021).

PD is a recognizable neurodegenerative disorder with diverse causes and different clinical presentations characterized by motor and non-motor symptoms. Four cardinal features of PD can be grouped under the acronym TRAP: Tremor at rest, rigidity, akinesia (or bradykinesia), and postural instability (Jankovic, 2008). PD frequently presents with tremors, typically seen in one extremity. This tremor is slower (4-6 Hz) than a classic essential tremor (8-10 Hz) and is most prominent when the limb is in a repose posture. For some patients, the classic parkinsonian tremor is the only manifestation of the disease (tremor-predominant PD) (Hayes, 2019). Rigidity is characterized by increased resistance and can prevent muscles from stretching and relaxing as they should. Akinesia is a term used to describe the loss of ability to move muscles voluntarily, while bradykinesia means slowness of movement and can be expressed in different ways: reduction of automatic movements, difficulty initiating movements, general slowness in physical actions, the appearance of abnormal stillness or a decrease in facial expression (Bloem et al., 2021). Postural instability due to loss of postural reflexes is generally a manifestation of the late stages of PD and usually occurs after the onset of other clinical features (Jankovic, 2008).

Although motor features define the disorder, various non-motor features typically are seen (Pfeiffer, 2016), including autonomic dysfunction (e.g., constipation, bloating, nausea, and abdominal discomfort), psychiatric changes (e.g., depression and anxiety), sensory symptoms (e.g., anosmia occurs in as many as 90% of patients), sleep disturbances, and cognitive symptoms. Dementia can occur in an important number of patients with a prevalence close to 30% (Hanagasi et al., 2017).

Pathophysiology

PD has been associated with a loss or degeneration of the dopaminergic neurons in the *substantia nigra* as well as the presence of abnormal intraneuronal conglomerates of α-synuclein protein (Lewy bodies) (Hayes,

2019). PD's pathophysiology seems to result from the interaction of present Lewy Bodies, mitochondrial dysfunction, lysosomes or vesicle transport, synaptic transport issues, and neuroinflammation. The complex interaction of these mechanisms drives accelerated neuronal death of primarily dopaminergic neurons, involving both motor and non-motor circuits (Bloem et al., 2021).

Dopamine deficiency produces dysfunction in the striatum, leading to 1) Decreased activity in the direct pathway, from GABAergic striatal neurons to the internal segment of the globus pallidus (GPi) and *substantia nigra pars reticulata* (SNpr) and 2) Increased drive through the indirect pathway, particularly involving the external segment of the globus pallidus (GPe) and subthalamic nucleus (STN). Consequently, there is disruption of the activity in basal ganglia output structures such as GPi and SNpr, which in turn disrupts the activity in brain stem motor areas, including the pedunculopontine nucleus and the thalamocortical motor system (Hamani et al., 2016). This disruption is thought to be responsible for the difficulty in movement initiation and the poverty of motion, characteristic of PD (Figure 1).

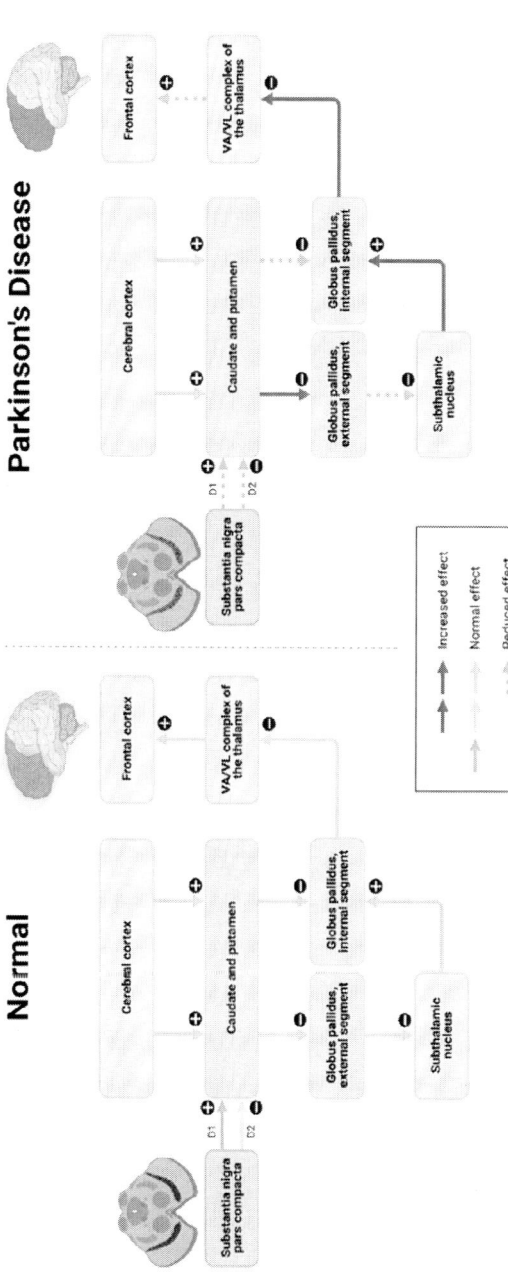

Figure 1. Pathophysiology of Parkinson's Disease. Under normal circumstances (left), the direct and indirect pathways of the basal ganglia produce an opposite excitatory and inhibitory effect, respectively, on the VA and VL nuclei of the thalamus, the balance of which determines the appropriate motor responses of the cerebral cortex. In addition, dopaminergic fibers from the substantia nigra pars compacta are distributed throughout the caudate nucleus and the putamen, exerting a modulatory action dependent on the type of receptor. Axons acting on neurons with D1 receptors have an excitatory effect on them; on the other hand, those that do so on neurons with D2 receptors are of the inhibitory type. As a consequence of PD (right), when the neurons of the substantia nigra are lost, the dopamine deficit in the caudate nucleus and the putamen causes an imbalance of the direct and indirect pathways, the result of which is an increase in the inhibition of the thalamus and therefore the cerebral cortex loses thalamic regulation. VA: Ventroanterior. VL: Ventrolateral. PD: Parkinson's Disease.

Treatment

Although there is currently no cure for PD, diverse treatments are used to ameliorate the symptoms. Dopaminergic pharmacotherapy is one of the main strategies; dopamine precursors, like Levodopa, are the most used effective medication for PD and are still the most potent. These allow the depleted number of dopaminergic neurons to produce more dopamine and alleviate symptoms (Hayes, 2019). Dopamine agonists such as pramipexole, ropinirole, and rotigotine are also used to stimulate dopaminergic receptors in the central nervous system (CNS), which alleviate PD symptoms (Table 1).

Table 1. Current medical treatment of Parkinson's Disease

Pharmacological group	Drug	Mechanism of action
Anticholinergics	Trihexyphenidyl Biperiden	Effective against tremor, otherwise they are limited efficacy. They have significant side effects
Adamantanes	Amantadine	It is an antiviral drug. As an antiparkinsonian drug, it seems to favor a dopaminergic response by releasing dopamine and inhibiting its reuptake
Dopamine agonists	Levodopa	The symptomatic treatment of choice. It is converted into dopamine by the action of DOPA-decarboxylase. It must be administered with a decarboxylase inhibitor such as carbidopa or benserazide to reduce this biotransformation outside the nervous system
Catechol-O-methyl-transferase inhibitors	Tolcapone Entacapone Opicapone	They are drugs that inhibit the peripheral metabolism of L-DOPA by Catechol-O-methyltransferase, which increases its bioavailability
Monoamine oxidase B inhibitors	Selegiline Rasagiline Safinamide	They are drugs that inhibit the peripheral metabolism of L-DOPA by mono amine oxidase B, which increases its bioavailability
Direct dopaminergic receptor agonists	Pramipexole Ropinirole Rotigotine Apomorphine	Unlike the previous ones, these drugs do not require biotransformation. They act on D2 and D3 receptors

Anticholinergic medications such as trihexyphenidyl and benztropine may be effective in decreasing rigidity, dystonia, and tremor. Antipsychotics are sometimes necessary to treat the symptoms of hallucination and paranoid delusions that occur in Parkinson's patients (Table 1). Most of the drugs available for the treatment of Parkinson's Disease act only at a symptomatic level, therefore delaying the evolution of the disorder. The search for new therapies is necessary.

Non-Pharmacological Interventions

Several features of PD do not respond adequately to optimal pharmacotherapy. This issue exacerbates with disease progression because neurodegeneration progressively involves non-dopaminergic brain areas. Moreover, dose-limiting side effects hamper the successful deployment of pharmacotherapy. This recognition fueled a drive toward an integrated multidisciplinary management approach, with potentially useful contributions from many different disciplines (Bloem et al., 2021).

In neurodegenerative diseases, it has so far not been possible to propose any causative therapy since the etiologies are still not well understood. The goal of neuroprotection is to either slow down or stop the processes leading to neuronal death in the CNS. The KD has been proposed as a palliative therapy for neurodegenerative diseases, such as Alzheimer's and Parkinson's (Wlodarek, 2019). In PD, animal and *in vitro* studies have demonstrated a beneficial effect of ketone bodies on the course of PD.

Ketogenic Diet Mechanisms

Under normal conditions, glucose is the CNS's main energy source. During ketosis, glucose reserves become insufficient for the brain's metabolism. Consequently, the liver converts fatty acids into ketone bodies (KB): acetoacetate (AcAc), β-hydroxybutyrate (BHB), and acetone (Figure 2) (Wlodarek, 2019). KB can cross the blood-brain barrier and are an efficient energy source for the brain, contributing to up to 60-70% of its energy needs (Morris et al., 2020; Zhu et al., 2022).

There are four different types of KD, each having a different macronutrient composition. In the classic ketogenic diet (CKD), the main sources of lipids are long-chain triglycerides (LCT), which are obtained from food. These represent approximately 80-90% of the total energy intake. The medium-chain triglyceride diet (MCTD) is more palatable. Fatty acids are primarily octanoic and decanoic, which are supplemented. These produce more ketones per calorie than LCT, allowing a higher carbohydrate and protein intake than CKD. Low glycemic index treatment (LGIT) also allows a higher carbohydrate and protein intake. Lipids contribute 45% of total daily calories. Focuses on the type of carbohydrates included in the diet, allowing only foods with a glycemic index of less than 50%. The modified Atkins diet (MAD) combines the KD and Atkins. Although it promotes a higher fat intake and allows for fewer carbohydrates, it is less restrictive since approximately 65% of total calories are obtained from fat (Barzegar et al., 2021).

Several studies have demonstrated that KD exerts a neuroprotective effect on PD, as it improves mitochondrial function and decreases oxidative stress (OS) and neuroinflammation. These play a crucial role in the onset and progression of the disease, although the underlying mechanisms are poorly understood (Zhu et al., 2022; Morris et al., 2020). OS occurs when there is an overproduction of reactive oxygen species (ROS). This imbalance causes alterations in dopamine metabolism and mitochondrial dysfunction (Włodarek, 2019) In contrast, the KB increase ATP yield and reduces ROS production, by enhancing nicotinamide adenine dinucleotide (NADH) oxidation and decreasing mitochondrial permeability transition (Wlodarek, 2019). Therefore, improving mitochondrial respiration (Zhu et al., 2022). Besides, the presence of KB enhances mitochondrial biogenesis (Wlodarek, 2019).

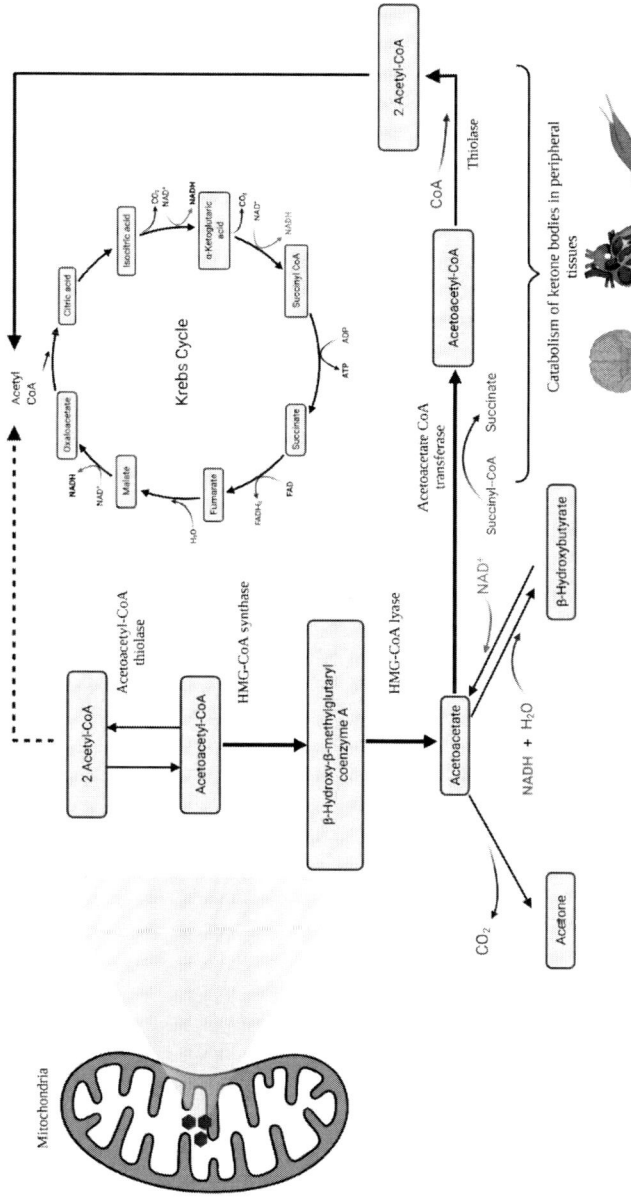

Figure 2. The synthesis of KBs begins with acetyl-CoA production from the beta-oxidation of fatty acids. Then, two acetyl-CoA molecules combine to form acetoacetyl-CoA. The latter is converted to AcAc, one of the primary ketone bodies, through the action of the thiolase enzyme. AcAc is released into the bloodstream and transported to peripheral tissues. In parallel, some of the AcAc is converted to BHB by the enzyme beta-hydroxybutyrate dehydrogenase, which represents another important ketone body. On the other hand, a small amount of AcAc is spontaneously converted to acetone, which is volatile and can be exhaled through breath or excreted in urine. These KBs, AcAc and BHB, are transported through the bloodstream from the liver to peripheral tissues, including the brain, heart, and muscles. In these tissues, are catabolized and converted back to acetyl-CoA, a molecule that can enter the citric acid cycle (Krebs cycle) and be used to produce ATP. AcAc: Acetoacetate. BHB: β-Hydroxybutirate. KBs: Ketone bodies.

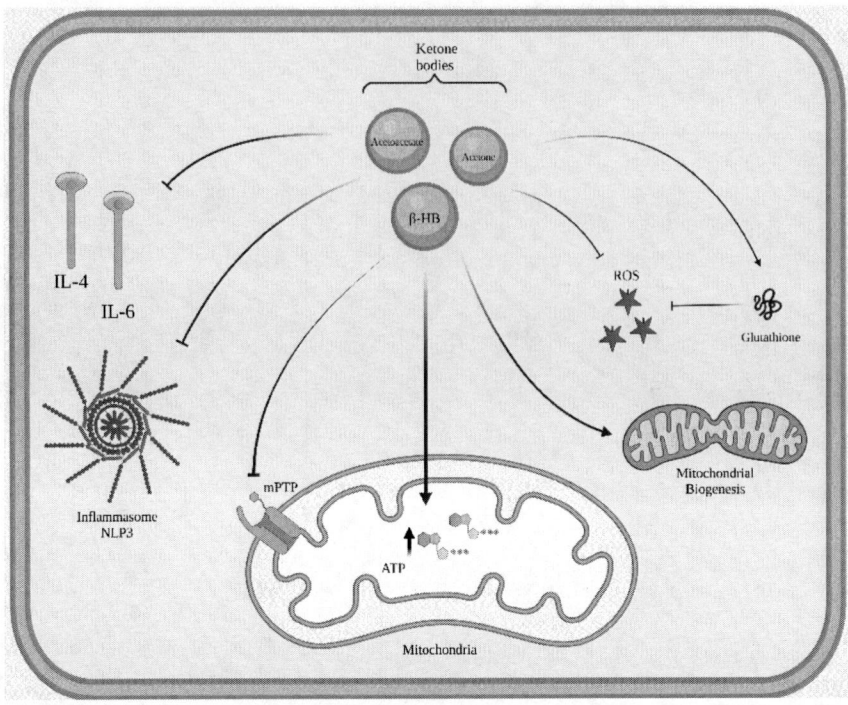

Figure 3. Neuroprotective effects of ketogenic diet on Parkinson's Disease. Neuroprotection in Parkinson's Disease by ketone bodies has been demonstrated in several ways. Ketone bodies have an inhibitory effect on inflammatory mediators such as IL-4, IL-6, and the inflammasome NLP3. Also, modulate the activity of mPTP. They may increase the expression of glutathione, which in turn can counteract ROS. And finally, ketone bodies stimulate mitochondrial biogenesis and improve ATP generation. mPTP: Mitochondrial permeability transition pore. ROS: Reactive oxygen species.

Additionally, a potential antioxidant effect of the KD has been reported. A study conducted with animals showed higher levels of glutathione peroxidase (GPx) in the hippocampus of rats fed a KD (Ziegler et al., 2003). Another recent study in children with epilepsy found higher levels of glutathione (GSH) after an intervention with KD (Napolitano et al., 2020). Further research has shown that KD decreases pro-inflammatory cytokines, such as IL-4, IL-6 and TNFα, therefore, it should prevent dopaminergic neuron degeneration (Yang and Cheng, 2010). Particularly, BHB has been reported to decrease neuroinflammation by inhibiting the expression of the inflammasome NLP3 (Figure 3). An early study by Kashiwaya et al. (2000), found that BHB acts *in vitro* as a neuroprotective agent against the toxicity of 1-methyl-4-phenyl-1,2,3,6-tetrahydropyridine (MPTP) on dopaminergic pathway.

Moreover, insulin resistance and a decreased glucose metabolism in the brain are risk factors implicated in the development of PD (Krikorian et al., 2019). During ketosis, carbohydrate restriction improves insulin and glucose levels (Krikorian et al., 2019), leading to enhanced cognitive function and neuron survival (Morris et al., 2020). Krikorian et al. (2012) observed that a short-term KD intervention decreased insulin resistance and improved glucose levels, leading to better cognitive performance in older adults with mild cognitive impairment. Recently, there has been increasing interest in the relationship between the gut microbiome and the pathogenesis of several diseases. Studies have found that KD can exert beneficial changes in the microbiota composition, including an increase in *Akkermansia Muciniphila* abundance. (Zhu et al., 2022). However, most studies have been carried out in animal models and there is still no evidence on the effect of KD on the intestinal microbiota of patients with PD.

Evidence of the Ketogenic Diet on PD's Symptoms

Although there is little evidence that demonstrates the positive effects of KD on PD, some studies have observed improvements in motor and non-motor symptoms. Table 2 shows the main findings of diverse patients and animal model studies.

Table 2. Studies that had assessed the effects of the ketogenic diet on Parkinson's disease symptoms

Author, year	Study design	Sample size	Outcomes
VanItallie et al., 2005	Patients with PD volunteered to maintain a KD for 28 days. The UPDRS were applied at baseline and after 28 days	n = 7 PD patients	With 2 exceptions, the participants adhered to the KD. The authors observed a 43.4% decrease in UPDRS score. The main symptoms improved were resting tremors, freezing, balance, gait, mood, and energy level. Unfortunately, this study did not have a control group to test the placebo effect.

Table 2. (Continued)

Author, year	Study design	Sample size	Outcomes
Krikorian et al., 2019	Nutritional intervention for patients with mild cognitive impairment associated with PD. Patients were randomly assigned to a High-carbohydrate diet or a low carbohydrate ketogenic regime. For all participants, cognitive performance, motor function, and anthropometric and metabolic parameters were measured.	n = 14, divided into 2 groups: Ketogenic groups n = 7 High-carbohydrate groups n = 7	Patients who received the KD demonstrated improvement in cognitive performance (lexical access, memory, and reduced interference in memory) along with reduced body weight and increased circulating BHB. However, no effects were observed in motor function.
Phillips et al., 2018	A pilot randomized study with PD patients randomly assigned to a low-fat or a ketogenic diet plan. The MDS-UPDRS were applied to all participants weekly, and weight and blood measures (HbA1C, triglycerides, HDL, LDL, total cholesterol, and CRP) were also assessed	n = 47 patients divided into two groups: Low-fat group initially n = 23; completed n = 22 KD group initially n = 24 completed n = 18	Both groups decreased their MDS-UPDRS relative to baseline. But the ketogenic group decreased more (41% of improvement) in Part 1 of the scale (nonmotor daily living experiences) than the low-fat group (11% of improvement).
Koyuncu et al., 2021	Clinical trial on PD patients with voice quality impairment. Patients were randomly assigned to a regular diet group or a KD group. The VHI test was applied at baseline and after the 3-months intervention.	n = 74 patients divided into two groups: Regular diet initially n = 37, completed n = 34 KD initially n = 37, completed n = 34	No significant differences in the VHI test between groups were observed at baseline. However, after the 3-months treatment, a significant improvement was found in the KD groups, but not in the regular diet.
Animal Models			
Shaafi et al., 2016	An experimental study with a rat model of 6-OHDA-induced PD. The study includes control for diet (regular vs ketogenic), surgery (sham groups vs lesion), and medication (pramipexole vs no drug). Motor function was assessed by three tests: bar test, beam traversal task test, and cylinder task.	n = 56 male Wistar rats divided into seven, 8 rat groups: Healthy Groups: Normal diet Sham surgical KD 6-OHDA-induced PD groups: Normal diet KD Pramipexole and normal	In the healthy groups, no significant differences were found for any test. The PD groups had worst performance than the healthy groups. Among the Parkinsonian rats, better results were observed in the ketogenic groups compared to the normal diet group. The KD was significantly effective in promoting motor functions in Parkinsonian animals

Author, year	Study design	Sample size	Outcomes
		Pramipexole and Ketogenic Diet	and at the same time, enhanced the therapeutic effects of concomitantly administered pramipexole.
Kuter et al., 2021	An experimental study with a rat model of 6-OHDA-induced PD. The study includes control for diet and surgery (sham groups). Animals were kept on the stringent KD for 3 weeks before and 4 weeks after the brain operation. Locomotor activity, neuron count, dopaminergic terminal density, dopamine level, and turnover were analyzed at three time-points post-lesion, up to 4 weeks after the operation.	n = Not specified Regular diet + sham Regular diet + lesion KD + sham KD + lesion	Despite long-term hyperketonemia pre- and post-lesion, the KD did not protect against 6-OHDA-induced dopaminergic neuron lesions. The KD only tended to improve locomotor activity and normalize DA turnover in the striatum. Rats fed 7 weeks in total with a restrictive KD maintained normoglycemia, and neither gluconeogenesis nor glycogenolysis in the liver was responsible for this effect.

Side Effects

During the transition to ketosis, symptoms such as fatigue, irritability, headaches, nausea, emesis, dehydration, diarrhea, insomnia, and hypoglycemia are common. Adequate hydration and electrolyte intake can help reduce these side effects. Nonetheless, these are normally resolved after a few days or weeks once the organism has adapted to the metabolic changes (Włodarek, 2019). On the other hand, long-term side effects include nausea, emesis, abdominal pain, decreased appetite, and constipation. These are mainly caused by low tolerance to high lipid intake, and depending on severity, decrease the compliance with the diet (Włodarek, 2019; Zhu et al., 2022).

Adverse Effects

Long-term adverse effects should also be taken into consideration. KD increases the risk of cardiovascular disease (altered lipid profile, increased uric acid levels), nephrolithiasis, liver dysfunction, neuropathy, anemia, and osteoporosis. Therefore, these conditions should be monitored (Zhu et al., 2022; Phillips et al., 2018). Furthermore, it is known that patients who follow KD tend to decrease their caloric intake and consequently lose weight, mainly because the diet is poorly tolerated and the high lipid intake increases satiety. The above is a matter of special concern in patients with PD, as they already are at risk of malnutrition and sarcopenia (Włodarek, 2019).

Long-Term Safety

Most clinical evidence on the improvement of non-motor and motor symptoms in patients with PD are studies with small samples and short-duration interventions. Therefore, the long-term effectiveness and safety of KD remain uncertain (Zhu et al., 2022; Wlodarek, 2019). Furthermore, compliance with the KD could be demanding to maintain due to restrictiveness, low tolerance, and unpleasant side effects of the nutritional regime.

Conclusion

The evidence on the beneficial effects of KD in neurodegenerative diseases is promising. Some consequences have been observed in both clinical trials and animal models of PD: it has been found that KD can help improve motor symptoms, such as decreased resting tremor, balance, freezing, locomotor activity. Additionally, non-motor symptoms, including improvements in cognition (mainly memory), activities of daily living, and even the voice impairment typically associated with PD, have been observed to decrease after a KD. Therefore, KD could be a palliative and complementary treatment for patients suffering from PD. Although the exact mechanisms behind these effects are still unknown, it has been hypothesized that ketosis causes structural and functional cellular and synaptic changes that reinforce bioenergy (enhancing mitochondrial function) and resistance to OS. Nevertheless, in addition to the limited evidence to support the effects of KD on PD's symptom improvement, many limitations may impede the representative nature of the research mentioned in this chapter, such as small samples, lack of control groups (especially for human studies) and therefore, possible placebo effects. In summary, further research is needed on both the effects of KD and the underlying mechanisms.

Disclaimer

None.

References

Barzegar, M., Afghan, M., Tarmahi, V., Behtari, M., Rahimi Khamaneh, S., & Raeisi, S. (2021). Ketogenic diet: overview, types, and possible anti-seizure mechanisms. *Nutritional Neuroscience*, *24*(4), 307–316. https://doi.org/10.1080/1028415X.2019.1627769

Bloem, B. R., Okun, M. S., & Klein, C. (2021). Parkinson's disease. *The Lancet*, *397*(10291), 2284–2303. https://doi.org/10.1016/S0140-6736(21)00218-X

Hamani, C., Lozano, A. M., Mazzone, P. A. M., Moro, E., Hutchison, W., Silburn, P. A., Zrinzo, L., Alam, M., Goetz, L., Pereira, E., Rughani, A., Thevathasan, W., Aziz, T., Bloem, B. R., Brown, P., Chabardes, S., Coyne, T., Foote, K., Garcia-Rill, E., … Krauss, J. K. (2016). Pedunculopontine Nucleus Region Deep Brain Stimulation in Parkinson Disease: Surgical Techniques, Side Effects, and Postoperative Imaging. *Stereotactic and Functional Neurosurgery*, *94*(5), 307–319. https://doi.org/10.1159/000449011

Hanagasi, H. A., Tufekcioglu, Z., & Emre, M. (2017). Dementia in Parkinson's disease. *Journal of the Neurological Sciences*, *374*, 26–31. https://doi.org/10.1016/j.jns.2017.01.012

Hayes, M. T. (2019). Parkinson's Disease and Parkinsonism. *The American Journal of Medicine*, *132*(7), 802–807. https://doi.org/10.1016/j.amjmed.2019.03.001

Jankovic, J. (2008). Parkinson's disease: clinical features and diagnosis. *Journal of Neurology, Neurosurgery & Psychiatry*, *79*(4), 368–376. https://doi.org/10.1136/jnnp.2007.131045

Kashiwaya, Y., Takeshima, T., Mori, N., Nakashima, K., Clarke, K., & Veech, R. L. (2000). <scp>d</scp> -β-Hydroxybutyrate protects neurons in models of Alzheimer's and Parkinson's disease. *Proceedings of the National Academy of Sciences*, *97*(10), 5440–5444. https://doi.org/10.1073/pnas.97.10.5440

Koyuncu, H., Fidan, V., Toktas, H., Binay, O., & Celik, H. (2021). Effect of ketogenic diet versus regular diet on voice quality of patients with Parkinson's disease. *Acta Neurologica Belgica*, *121*(6), 1729–1732. https://doi.org/10.1007/s13760-020-01486-0

Krikorian, R., Shidler, M. D., Summer, S. S., Sullivan, P. G., Duker, A. P., Isaacson, R. S., & Espay, A. J. (2019). Nutritional ketosis for mild cognitive impairment in Parkinson's disease: A controlled pilot trial. *Clinical Parkinsonism & Related Disorders*, *1*, 41–47. https://doi.org/10.1016/j.prdoa.2019.07.006

Kuter, K. Z., Olech, L., Glowacka, U., & Paleczna, M. (2021). Increased Beta-Hydroxybutyrate Level Is Not Sufficient for the Neuroprotective Effect of Long-

Term Ketogenic Diet in an Animal Model of Early Parkinson's Disease. Exploration of Brain and Liver Energy Metabolism Markers. *International Journal of Molecular Sciences*, *22*(14), 7556. https://doi.org/10.3390/ijms22147556

Morris, G., Maes, M., Berk, M., Carvalho, A. F., & Puri, B. K. (2020). Nutritional ketosis as an intervention to relieve astrogliosis: Possible therapeutic applications in the treatment of neurodegenerative and neuroprogressive disorders. *European Psychiatry*, *63*(1), e8. https://doi.org/10.1192/j.eurpsy.2019.13

Najmi, S., Shaafi, S., Aliasgharpour, H., Mahmoudi, J., Sadigh-Etemad, S., Farhoudi, M., & Baniasadi, N. (2016). Iranian Journal of Neurology © 2016 The efficacy of the ketogenic diet on motor functions in Parkinson's disease: A rat model. In *Iran J Neurol* (Vol. 15, Issue 2). http://ijnl.tums.ac.ir

Napolitano, A., Longo, D., Lucignani, M., Pasquini, L., Rossi-Espagnet, M. C., Lucignani, G., Maiorana, A., Elia, D., De Liso, P., Dionisi-Vici, C., & Cusmai, R. (2020). The Ketogenic Diet Increases In Vivo Glutathione Levels in Patients with Epilepsy. *Metabolites*, *10*(12), 504. https://doi.org/10.3390/metabo10120504

National Parkinson Foundation. (n.d.). *"What is Parkinson?" Parkinson Foundation.* . 2022.

Paoli, A., Bianco, A., Damiani, E., & Bosco, G. (2014). Ketogenic Diet in Neuromuscular and Neurodegenerative Diseases. *BioMed Research International*, *2014*, 1–10. https://doi.org/10.1155/2014/474296

Pfeiffer, R. F. (2016). Non-motor symptoms in Parkinson's disease. *Parkinsonism & Related Disorders*, *22*, S119–S122. https://doi.org/10.1016/j.parkreldis.2015.09.004

Phillips, M. C. L., Murtagh, D. K. J., Gilbertson, L. J., Asztely, F. J. S., & Lynch, C. D. P. (2018). Low-fat versus ketogenic diet in Parkinson's disease: A pilot randomized controlled trial. *Movement Disorders*, *33*(8), 1306–1314. https://doi.org/10.1002/mds.27390

VanItallie, T. B., Nonas, C., Di Rocco, A., Boyar, K., Hyams, K., & Heymsfield, S. B. (2005). Treatment of Parkinson disease with diet-induced hyperketonemia: A feasibility study. *Neurology*, *64*(4), 728–730. https://doi.org/10.1212/01.WNL.0000152046.11390.45

Włodarek, D. (2019). Role of Ketogenic Diets in Neurodegenerative Diseases (Alzheimer's Disease and Parkinson's Disease). *Nutrients*, *11*(1), 169. https://doi.org/10.3390/nu11010169

Yang, X., & Cheng, B. (2010). Neuroprotective and Anti-inflammatory Activities of Ketogenic Diet on MPTP-induced Neurotoxicity. *Journal of Molecular Neuroscience*, *42*(2), 145–153. https://doi.org/10.1007/s12031-010-9336-y

Zhu, H., Bi, D., Zhang, Y., Kong, C., Du, J., Wu, X., Wei, Q., & Qin, H. (2022). Ketogenic diet for human diseases: the underlying mechanisms and potential for clinical implementations. *Signal Transduction and Targeted Therapy*, *7*(1), 11. https://doi.org/10.1038/s41392-021-00831-w

Ziegler, D. R., Ribeiro, L. C., Hagenn, M., Siqueira, Ionara R., Araújo, E., Torres, I. L. S., Gottfried, C., Netto, C. A., & Gonçalves, C. (2003). Ketogenic diet increases glutathione peroxidase activity in rat hippocampus. *Neurochemical Research*, *28*(12), 1793–1797. https://doi.org/10.1023/A:1026107405399

Chapter 3

The Ketogenic Diet and Alzheimer's Disease

Ernesto Ochoa[1]
Fernando Gatica[1]
Zayra Morales[1]
Héctor Romo-Parra[2]
Luis Antonio Marín-Castañeda[1,3]
and Carmen Rubio[*]

[1]Departamento de Neurofisiología, Instituto Nacional de Neurología y Neurocirugía, Manuel Velasco Suárez, Mexico City, Mexico
[2]Centro de Investigación en Psicología, Facultad de Psicología, Universidad Iberoamericana, Mexico City, Mexico
[3]Facultad Mexicana de Medicina, Universidad La Salle, Mexico City, Mexico

Abstract

Alzheimer's disease is a form of dementia characterized by progressive loss of memory and other cortical functions. The causes that led to the development of this disease are unknown. However, some predisposing factors have been identified, such as age, genetics, and family history. Although it is not traditionally considered an inflammatory disease, there are inflammation-related processes that can be decisive in presenting this pathology. In addition, oxidative stress has been shown to be involved in pathogenesis. Coupled with the lack of response to conventional treatments, diet therapies have become attractive for new therapy approaches. The ketogenic diet has interesting properties due to its metabolic impact and has been shown to be effective in neurological

---

[*] Corresponding Author's Email: macaru4@yahoo.com.mx.

In: The Ketogenic Diet Reexamined
Editors: Leticia Granados-Rojas and Carmen Rubio
ISBN: 979-8-89113-543-7
© 2024 Nova Science Publishers, Inc.

disorders. Action mechanisms, inflammation, and oxidative stress represent important targets that could ameliorate the deleterious consequences of Alzheimer's disease.

Keywords: Alzheimer's disease, ketogenic diet, ketone bodies, inflammation, reactive oxygen species, mitochondria

Acronyms

AD	Alzheimer's disease
AMPA	α-amino-3-hydroxy-5-methyl-4-isoxazolepropionic acid
APOE	Apolipoprotein E
APP	Amyloid precursor protein
ATP	Adenosine triphosphate
Aβ	Amyloid β peptide
BBB	Blood-brain barrier
BDNF	Brain-derived neurotrophic factor
BHB	β-hydroxybutyrate
cAMP	Cyclic adenosine monophosphate
CNS	Central nervous system
GDNF	Glial cell line-derived neurotrophic factor
GLUT	Glucose transporter
HCA2	Hydroxycarboxylic acid 2
HCA2	Hydroxycarboxylic acid receptor 2
KB	Ketone bodies
KD	Ketogenic diet
mPTP	Mitochondrial permeability transition pore
NFκB	Nuclear factor kappa-light-chain-enhancer of activated B cells
NIACR1	Niacin receptor 1
NLRP3	NLR family pyrin domain containing 3
Nrf2	Nuclear factor erythroid 2-related factor 2
NSAID	Nonsteroidal anti-inflammatory drugs
NT-3	Neurotrophin 3
PPARγ	Peroxisome proliferator-activated receptor gamma
ROS	Reactive oxygen species
VEFG	Pro-angiogenic factors

Introduction

Alzheimer's disease (AD), the most common form of dementia, is a syndrome of progressive cognitive deterioration that affects more than 30 million people worldwide (Villemagne et al., 2013). Despite extensive research, its etiology remains unclear. Several mechanisms have been described, such as genetic predisposition, mitochondrial dysfunction, inflammation, oxidative stress, insulin resistance, and impaired glucose utilization in the brain (Lane et al., 2018). AD is distinguished by the presence of a large number of deposits of a protein fragment known as amyloid β-peptide (Aβ) in the brain, which accumulates in the spaces between nerve cells. On the other hand, tangles are twisted fibers of the Tau protein that accumulate inside the cell. These pathological hallmarks lead to neuronal destruction and hypometabolism leading to a decline in cognitive functions (Winkler et al., 2015).

In the realm of AD treatment, it is evident that not all patients respond adequately to conventional therapies. This observation has prompted a search for alternative strategies that could play a role in the management of this disease. Among these potential approaches, the ketogenic diet (KD) has attracted considerable attention. In addition to the fat content derived from KD, this diet can serve as an alternative fuel for neurons because they lose the ability to break down glucose for energy (Gasior et al., 2006). This regime has also been shown to be beneficial in those cases of drug-resistant AD.

KD is characterized by a reduced carbohydrate intake compared to conventional diets, thus reducing the energy required for the biochemical and genetic mechanisms involved in AD. Although research on the therapeutic potential of diet interventions in AD have remained somewhat limited since 1990, substantial interest has grown in the use of KD to treat drug-resistant AD. It has been found that nearly half of patients treated with KD have reported an improvement in symptoms. Chronic ketosis is the central underlying mechanism, promoting synaptic stabilization, increasing brainenergy reserve, and improving mitochondrial function and biogenesis, as well as inhibiting apoptotic factors, reducing inflammation and the production of oxidative stress (Veech, 2004). Consequently, in this chapter, we will review some of the mechanisms underlying KD in the context of AD treatment.

General Aspects of Ketogenic Diet and Alzheimer's Disease

Neuropathology of AD encompasses diffuse deposits of amyloid plaques that contain Aβ isoforms Aβ1-40 and Aβ1-42, along with Tau protein. Both accumulate and cause neurotoxicity in areas of the brain responsible for memory and cognitive processes, including the limbic system, subcortical structures, and the neocortex, with progressive synaptic dysfunction in addition to neuronal loss (Takahashi et al., 2017; Rusek et al., 2019).

The brain relies on glucose as its main source of energy for neurons, which is facilitated by glucose transporters (GLUTs). In AD, there is a reduction in these transporters, leading to decreased glucose uptake and inefficient glycolysis, both of which are associated with progressive cognitive impairment (Winkler et al., 2015). As a result, an alternative source of energy is the ketone bodies (KB), including β-hydroxybutyrate (BHB), acetone, and acetoacetate. These KB produce more energy per unit of oxygen compared to glucose (Fukao et al., 2004). KB are derived from the breakdown of fatty acids through lipolysis. Given the promising effects of diets with high lipid content, such as KD, researchers have explored their potential to improve neuronal metabolism, especially their antioxidant and anti-inflammatory effects, and their benefit on cognitive processes (Veech, 2004) (Figure 1).

KDs have been used for more than 100 years to treat drug-resistant neurological diseases such as epilepsy. The exploration of other brain disorders that can offer neuroprotective effects has gained significant attention in recent research (Huttenlocher, 1976). They are characterized by low carbohydrate intake and high lipid consumption. A typical KD contains between 70% to 80% fats, 10% to 20% proteins, (enough for growth and development), and 5% to 10% carbohydrates (Gasior et al., 2006). When dietary carbohydrates are limited, the brain transitions to its secondary energy source, KB. This shift triggers a change in glucose metabolism towards the metabolism of fatty acids, reducing the production of glycolytic adenosine triphosphate (ATP) and increasing mitochondrial oxidation's ATP production. This metabolic state is favorable, offering protection against neuronal loss attributed to apoptosis and necrosis (Cahill, 2006).

Thus, KD is considered a form of metabolic therapy and prevention by providing alternative energy substrates in neurodegenerative diseases such as AD. KD administered for a long period of time is known to reduce the accumulation of Aβ and Tau protein in the brain while mitigating their toxicity (Broom et al., 2019). Furthermore, KD positively impacts cognitive functions by promoting angiogenesis and increasing capillary density, thus improving learning and memory skills (Vinciguerra et al., 2020).

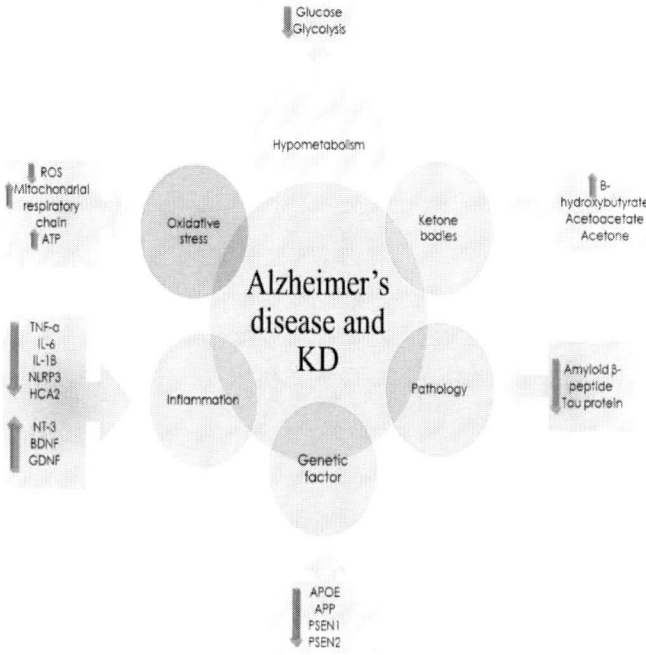

Figure 1. Mechanisms involved in the pathogenesis of Alzheimer's disease and how the ketogenic diet (KD) acts on each one. The effect of the ketogenic diet is exemplified with arrows, ↓: decreased, ↑: increased. ROS: reactive oxygen species. HCA2: hydroxycarboxylic acid 2. NT-3: neurotrophin 3. BDNF: brain-derived neurotrophic factor. GDNF: glial cell line-derived neurotrophic factor.

In the first days of the diet, glucose concentrations decrease as well as the insulin-glucagon ratio. After three or four days, the reduction of carbohydrate intake leads to a decrease in glucogenesis, and liver glucose reserves become insufficient to meet the body's metabolic demand, especially in the nervous system. Consequently, the body seeks an alternative energy source that is provided by KB (Barnard et al., 2014). KB concentrations under normal conditions are less than 0.3 mmol/L, when this concentration exceeds 4 mmol / L, they become a significant energy source for the brain (Dhillon & Gupta, 2024). Increased KB production and subsequent reduction in blood glucose concentration are key factors that contribute to the therapeutic effects of KD.

KB also shows neuroprotective effects by increasing the efficiency of the mitochondrial respiratory chain through the intensification of ATP synthesis. Additionally, it reduces the production of reactive oxygen species (ROS) by decreasing pro-inflammatory and pro-apoptotic molecules, and by boosting the levels of neuroprotective factors such as neurotrophins (Maalouf et al., 2009).

Despite its potential benefits, KD requires significant changes in dietary habits, which poses a challenge for long-term adherence. Compliance with the diet can complicate its overall effectiveness, and various adverse effects have been reported. Among the most observed in Alzheimer's patients undergoing a KD are irritability, fatigue, insomnia, headache, constipation, or diarrhea, and other less common such as pancreatitis, hypertriglyceridemia, decreased appetite, and hypoglycemia (Włodarek, 2019). Long-term effects, such as decreased bone density, vitamin or mineral deficiencies, and anemia have also been reported (Paoli et al., 2014).

Pathogenesis of Alzheimer's Disease

Among neurodegenerative diseases, a series of events coexist that culminate in the progressive loss of neurons and a subsequent decline in brain activity. In the case of AD, two key actions underpin its pathogenesis (Figure 2):

a) *β-amyloid* and amyloidogenic pathway: The initiation of AD is attributed to β-amyloid, wherein the amyloid precursor protein (APP), a transmembrane protein, undergoes enzymatic cleavage. Under physiological conditions, it is cleaved by two enzymes: α-secretase and γ-secretase. This pathway is known as the nonamyloidogenic pathway and produces soluble peptides that are not harmful to neurons. The α-secretase divides the polypeptide into two similar parts, while the γ-secretase divides it through the transmembrane domain. If the excision of APP occurs by the β-secretase or β-amyloid converting enzyme, followed by the γ-secretase, the resulting product will be Aβ, which is an insoluble peptide. This pathway is known as the amyloidogenic pathway (Reiss et al., 2018).

In the early stages, the aggregation of Aβ peptides forms oligomers in the extracellular space, and later amyloid plaques are built to interfere with the central nervous system (CNS) function. Microscopically, these lesions are observed as spherical plaques with dilated extensions derived from dystrophic axons around a central amyloid nucleus. However, it should be noted that activated microglia and reactive astrocytes are also found, which demonstrates the involvement of the immune response in the pathogenesis of this disease (Selkoe, 2001).

b) *Tau protein and neurofibrillary tangles.* Tau protein typically resides within the microtubule network of axons. In AD, the kinase is hyperactivated responsible for phosphorylation of Tau protein, leading to its relocation to somatodendritic areas. As a result, there is an incorrect union with the rest of the microtubule proteins, which leads to microtubule instability and cell death. It is histologically observed as neurofibrillary tangles (paired helical bundles within the neuronal cytoplasm that displace or surround the nucleus). These neurofibrillary tangles persist in the tissue even after neuronal death (Ballard et al., 2011).

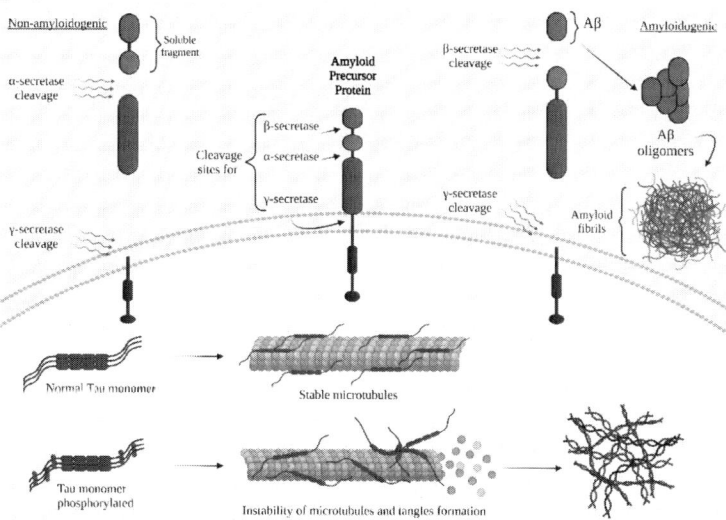

Figure 2. Pathological findings in Alzheimer's disease. Under normal conditions, the amyloid precursor protein is cleaved by two enzymes, α-secretase and γ-secretase in the non-amyloidogenic pathway, which generates harmless soluble peptides.
However, in the amyloidogenic pathway, when β-secretase and γ-secretase cleavage occurs, amyloid-β is released, forming amyloid fibrils and amyloid plaques. The Tau protein contributes to the stabilization of microtubules, but in a hyperphosphorylated state, the opposite occurs, leading to tangles formation and cell death. Aβ: Amyloid-β protein.

Neuroinflammation

Inflammation consists of a response to tissue damage to preserve cellular homeostasis. 2000 years ago, Cornelius Celsus described four cardinal manifestations of inflammation: blush, tumor, heat, and pain, which are four signs and symptoms consistent with cellular alterations of inflamed tissues. In 1858, Rudolph Virchow added a fifth cardinal sign: loss of function (Medzhitov, 2010).

The representative cell of the mononuclear phagocyte system in the CNS is the microglia or the Rio-Hortega cell. Its activation is the key determinant of neuroinflammation. Neurons and the rest of neuroglia also play an important role (Forloni & Balducci, 2018). When damage is detected in the CNS, microglial cells are activated, modifying their morphology and becoming mobile to target the lesion and carry out their phagocytic action. Additionally, the M1 phenotype can express pro-inflammatory molecules (TNF-α, IL-1β, IL-6) to promote the immune response and eliminate what causes damage (Holmes, 2013). If it is necessary to suppress excessive response or repair damaged tissue, the M2 phenotype can secrete IL-10 and proangiogenic factors (VEFG) (Tang & Le, 2016). Another factor that induces microglial activity is ATP levels. Under energy stress, neurons can release ATP, which attracts and activates microglia, with consequent cell migration mediated by chemoreceptors (P2Y12R and P2X4R). Subsequently, these alterations can activate adhesion molecules known as integrins. Their activity achieves the reorganization of the actin cytoskeleton (Yang & Zhou, 2019).

Physiologically, in healthy adults, microglial cells protect neurons from toxic damage from APP thanks to their phagocytic action that eliminates oligomers and prevents their accumulation (Hansen et al., 2018). However, in chronic inflammatory states, such as obesity, microglial cells have been observed to induce hyperreactivity with the consequent release of pro-inflammatory cytokines and the dysfunction of phagocytic activity. The inflammatory state leads to instability of the axonal cytoskeleton and the formation of dystrophic neurites with Aβ plaques that are not eliminated by phagocytes (O'Brien & Wong, 2011). These amyloid plaques perpetuate inflammation by releasing more cytokines such as TNF-α, IL-1β, in addition to ROS. Therefore, a vicious cycle of chronic inflammation is maintained and prolonged until the clinical manifestations of AD develop.

On the other hand, decreased microglial activity can also contribute to the development of AD. In older people, deterioration of the immune system is expected with the respective senescence of the phagocytes, which is evident in the greater propensity of older people to certain infectious and oncological diseases. In the case of microglia, the cellular changes that occur with aging are translated into dystrophic microglia which are also associated with neurofibrillary degeneration, important for the temporal lobe. This microglial hypoactivity event may be the final trigger for AD (Caldeira et al., 2014).

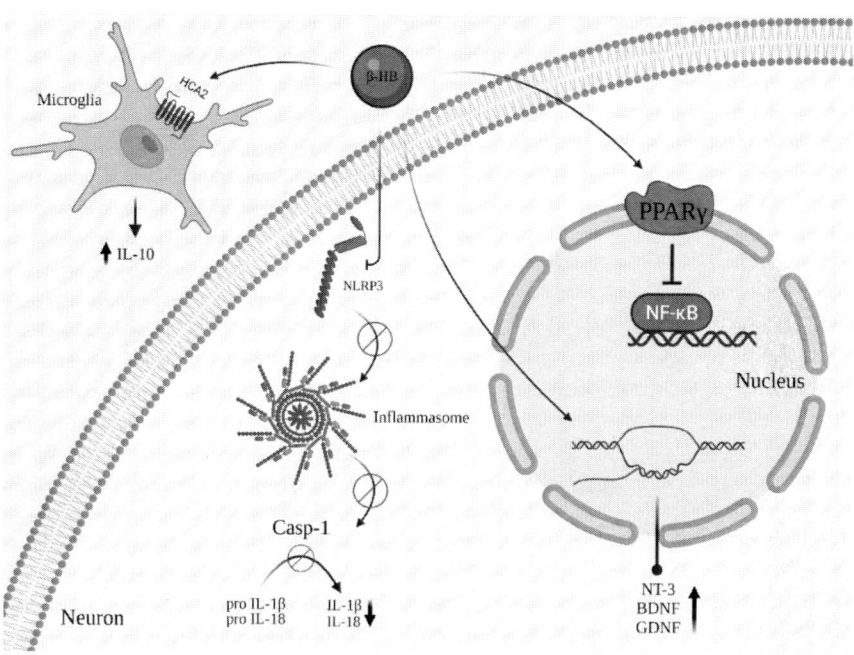

Figure 3. Ketogenic Diet effects. BHB has important anti-inflammatory and neuroprotective actions. In microglial cells, BHB binds to the HCA2 membrane receptor, which induces the expression of IL-10. In the cytoplasm, BHB is capable of inhibiting NLRP3, thus inhibiting the synthesis of the inflammasome protein complex, preventing the conversion of IL-1β and IL-18 from their precursors pro IL-1β and pro IL-18, respectively. The neuroprotective effect of BHB occurs through increased gene transcription of NT-3, BDNF, and GDNF. At the nuclear level, BHB activates the PPARγ receptor, thus inhibiting the nuclear expression of NFκB. β-HB: β-hydroxybutyrate. HCA2: Hydroxycarboxylic acid receptor 2. NLRP3: NLR family pyrin domain containing 3. NT-3: Neurotrophin-3. BDNF: Brain-derived neurotrophic factor. GDNF: Glial cell-derived neurotrophic factor. PPARγ: Peroxisome proliferator-activated receptor gamma. NFκB: nuclear factor kappa-light-chain-enhancer of activated B cells.

Thus, in the evolution of AD, microglial cells participate in two phases: 1) an early phase of microglial hyperactivity with excessive tissue damage; 2) a late phase of microglial senescence with minimal efficient phagocytic activity. The benefit of non-steroidal anti-inflammatory drugs (NSAIDs) in the early stages of AD is consistent, as the objective is to stop excessive inflammation. However, there is an association between the use of NSAIDs in the late stages and deterioration of function (Nazem et al., 2015). KD provides favorable effects in the prevention and treatment of AD from certain target molecules related to inflammation due to the production of KB, especially BHB (Figure 3).

a) *Hydroxycarboxylic acid receptor 2 (HCA2).* Also called niacin receptor 1 (NIACR1) or GPR109A and consists of a G-protein-coupled receptor, its agonists are BHB, butyric acid, and nicotinic acid or vitamin B3. HCA2 is expressed in microglia and its activation results in decreased inflammatory activity. This therapeutic target has already been used in other neurological diseases such as multiple sclerosis, in which monomethyl fumarate, an HCA2 agonist, has been shown to reduce inflammation in other autoimmune diseases (Offermanns, 2017).

b) *NLR family pyrin domain containing 3 (NLRP3).* Another target of ketones is an intracellular complex known as an inflammasome, of which NLRP3 has been described. NLRP3 regulates the activation of caspase-1 and thus, the release of IL-1 and IL-18 into extracellular space. This event is triggered by cathepsin B, released by the phagolysosome that phagocytosed the Aβ. Interest in cathepsin B in AD has grown in recent years (Kelley et al., 2019).

c) *PPAR γ – NFκB.* The fatty acids contributed by KD are endogenous ligands of the peroxisome proliferator-activated gamma receptor (PPARγ), which has positive effects on the regulation of macronutrient metabolism and negative consequences on the production of inflammatory cytokines. Furthermore, the nuclear factor kappa-light-chain-enhancer of activated B cells (NFκB) controls several genes involved in inflammation that may be related to the pathogenesis of AD, therefore its negative regulation is another beneficial effect of KD on AD via PPARγ (Nolte et al., 1998).

d) *Neurotrophins.* Neurotrophins are proteins that belong to the family of growth factors that favor the survival of neurons. Both by inhibiting apoptosis and by allowing cell growth and differentiation. KD has been shown to induce certain neurotrophins such as neurotrophin-3 (NT-3), brain-derived neurotrophic factor (BDNF), and glial cell line-derived neurotrophic factor (GDNF). In addition, KD can help to express certain molecules that favor correct protein folding known as chaperones (Rusek et al., 2019).

Neuroinflammation is also present in infectious diseases such as meningitis, encephalitis, and brain abscesses. Similarly, inflammatory responses have been found in other neurodegenerative diseases including dementia, movement disorders, epilepsy, and neuropsychiatric diseases such as anxiety, depression, and schizophrenia (Bostock et al., 2017; Wlodarek, 2019). This is an opportunity for the implementation of KD in other neurological and systemic pathologies.

Reactive Oxygen Species and Mitochondria

Among the pathological findings in AD, in addition to the accumulation of Aβ and neurofibrillary tangles, metabolic changes that affect mitochondria and glucose homeostasis have also been identified (Swerdlow, 2011). Impaired glycolysis and respiratory chain have been associated with a production and deposition of Aβ and neuronal death (McDonald & Cervenka, 2018; Wilkins & Swerdlow, 2017). Combined with oxidative stress, resulting from ROS produced in mitochondria, these are key factors associated with the molecular properties of KD (Manoharan et al., 2016) (Figure 4). The effects of KD on oxidative damage have been proven for several neurological disorders, mainly in epilepsy (Martin et al., 2016), where it has the same therapeutic targets by improving mitochondrial function and diminishing ROS damage. It seems that changing the metabolism from glucose to ketones is the mechanism by which KD works in neurological disorders. However, many of its properties are still being discovered.

Some studies have demonstrated the consequences of mitochondrial dysfunction in light of the pathogenesis of AD. Impaired glucose intake is associated with cognitive detriment not only in this pathology but also in aging (Swerdlow, 2011). Individuals with insulin resistance or genetically susceptible to AD have shown lower expression of GLUTs at the blood-brain barrier (BBB) with consequent cell starvation and the same cascade of events as for the AD findings (Carter et al., 2010; Verdile et al., 2015). Glucose intake impairment over a highly sensitive organ, as the brain may cause neural injury, supports the fact of an alternative dietary therapeutic for its treatment. Furthermore, the spectrum of damage encompasses hypometabolism, altered mitochondrial processes, and ROS generation, all of which are early findings in AD.

ROS are produced during oxidative phosphorylation even in the physiological state under tight equilibrium to avoid damaging their properties. Excess ROS can damage mitochondria and produce more ROS, resulting in dangerous self-perpetuating positive feedback. Mitochondria maintain a close balance in ROS production and, as observed, may be the cause and/or consequence of AD alterations. Poor antioxidant status and excessive ROS production have harmful effects on DNA, proteins, and lipids (Butterfield & Lauderback, 2002). In fact, patients with AD show these findings, both in peripheral tissues and in the brain, especially in the entorhinal cortex and hippocampus (Palmer & Burns, 1994; Baldeiras et al., 2008). Furthermore, Aβ interacts with β-adrenergic receptor, which, through the cyclic adenosine monophosphate (cAMP) protein kinase complex, phosphorylates subunit GluR1 from α-amino-3-hydroxy-5-methyl-4-isoxazolepropionic acid (AMPA) opening it and increasing the amount of calcium entry (Banke et al., 2000; Wang et al., 2010). Deleterious effects of calcium can go from mitochondrial damage with ROS production exacerbation to activation of programmed cell death.

Restriction of carbohydrates and a high intake of fats leads to alternative pathways of metabolism in the brain, capable of maintaining neuronal energy needs. Unlike carbohydrates, KB can pass through the BBB without the glucose transporter and reach mitochondria, avoiding glycolysis. The metabolic process of KD is more effective compared to carbohydrates. It restrains the imbalance between oxidant and antioxidant molecules in favor of the latter. This is because it activates the nuclear factor erythroid 2-related factor 2 (Nrf2), which in turn stimulates endogenous antioxidant systems such as glutathione, thioredoxin, peroxiredoxin, and heme oxygenase-1 (Kawai et al., 2011; Chorley et al., 2012). Another result of KB is the increased expression of uncoupling proteins, an inner mitochondrial membrane protein with several functions in energy metabolism (Sullivan et al., 2004), which leads to the transcription of many genes related to oxidative metabolism, as well as the down-regulation of ROS production by reducing the mitochondrial membrane potential (Harper et al., 2004; Rusek et al., 2019).

KB, particularly BHB, can activate mitochondrial ATP-sensitive potassium channels that work as calcium buffers, and therefore, inhibit mitochondrial permeability transition pore (mPTP), whose activity is related to cell death (Kim et al., 2015; Pinto et al., 2018). Additionally, in rats, the prevention of Aβ toxicity in hippocampal neurons has been demonstrated

(Kashiwaya et al., 2000). KD has the potential to inhibit the activation of AMPA receptors that, as we noticed, had deleterious results. Moreover, other components of some variants of KD, like decanoic acid, have interesting effects on neuroprotection not expressed by ketones. Decanoic acid is a PPARγ activator, a transcription factor that regulates genes associated with mitochondrial biogenesis (Hughes et al., 2014). Ultimately, enhanced mitochondrial renewal results in improved cellular energy and decreased Aβ deposition (Studzinski et al., 2008).

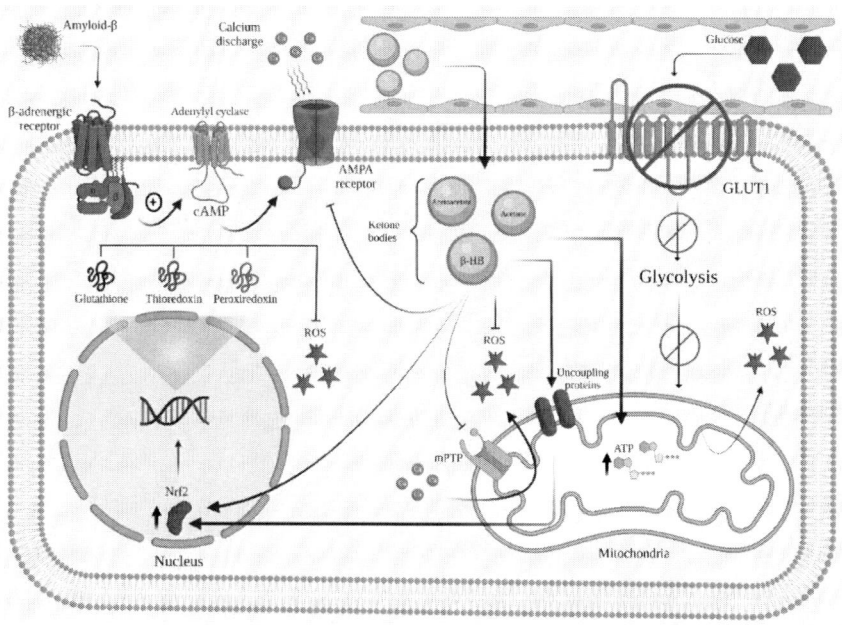

Figure 4. Molecular properties of ketone bodies (KB). KB has important antioxidant effects within the cell: Since neurons cannot use glucose as an energy source, KB provides a better amount of ATP in the respiratory chain of mitochondria. They have the ability to induce Nrf2 (alone or through uncoupling proteins) to stimulate the transcription of antioxidant systems such as glutathione, thioredoxin, or peroxiredoxin. Inhibit the expression of the mPTP. Block the influx of calcium from AMPA receptors (activated by amyloid-β through β-adrenergic receptors). ROS: reactive oxygen species. BHB: β-hydroxybutyrate. mPTP: mitochondrial permeability transition pore. Nrf2: nuclear factor erythroid 2-related factor 2. cAMP: cyclic adenosine monophosphate. AMPA: α-amino-3-hydroxy-5-methyl-4-isoxazolepropionic acid.

Notwithstanding the limited clinical studies of KD in AD, improved memory has been demonstrated in patients after treatment, and the correlation between KB in plasma and their cognitive performance reinforces KD as a potential adjuvant therapy (Henderson et al., 2009; Reger et al., 2004). Despite the lack of evidence in clinical studies, animal models in KD have been shown to improve mitochondrial function, suppress ROS, and attenuate Aβ accumulation (Van Der Auwera et al., 2005), which is a good basis for the investigation to continue.

Genetics

AD can be divided into two forms: monogenetic, in which a single genetic mutation can cause the disease, and polygenetic, in which susceptibility genes are found. Among the genes that have been investigated related to the risk of AD, the most associated is apolipoprotein E (APOE) in its form APOE3 (the most common), and APOE2, associated with the risk of early onset of the disease. So far, this gene is the most related to cerebral hypometabolism and in which the ketogenic diet could have an impact (Campion et al., 1999; Corder et al., 1993) (Figure 5).

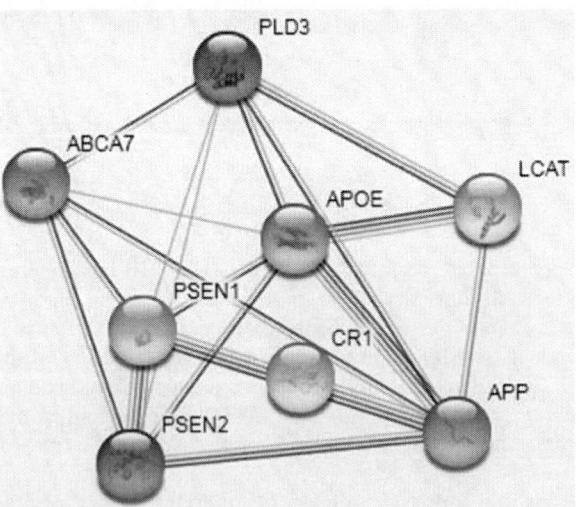

Figure 5. Genes found in patients with Alzheimer's disease. Until now, little is known about the function at the genetic level of the ketogenic diet (KD) in these patients; however, it has been possible to relate some of them, such as the APOE gene and APP, in which the KD reduces its expression.

Mutations in genes that encode proteins: APP, Presenilin 1 and Presenilin 2 cause the production of excessive amounts of Aβ (Goate et al., 1991; Tanzi & Bertram, 2005). Other genes related to AD are ABCA7 and PLD3, whose functions are not clear. However, their participation in the greater risk of suffering from the disease has been investigated. The CLUE gene has been explored to help regulate Aβ clearance from the brain in Alzheimer's patients. (Lleó et al., 2002). As already mentioned in this chapter, inflammation plays a crucial role in the pathology of the disease. Deficiency in the protein that generates the CR1 gene can contribute to chronic inflammation of the brain and the development of AD. (Kamboh, 2004). More research needs to be done on the impact of KD at the genetic level in AD patients.

Conclusion

KD stands as a compelling therapeutic option for various diseases. Although its establishment is not recent, the growing awareness of its underlying processes is a recent development. Given that AD is notoriously difficult to treat, the anticipation surrounding new treatments is entirely understandable. Dietary therapies have shown their effectiveness in addressing other disorders, raising hopes for similar results in AD. The mechanisms supporting this notion are being increasingly elucidated, and research progresses daily. The extent of research conducted will determine how we can implement KD more effectively in the future.

Disclaimer

None.

References

Baldeiras, I., Santana, I., Proença, M. T., Garrucho, M. H., Pascoal, R., Rodrigues, A., Duro, D., & Oliveira, C. R. (2008). Peripheral Oxidative Damage in Mild Cognitive Impairment and Mild Alzheimer's Disease. *Journal of Alzheimer's Disease*, *15*(1), 117–128. https://doi.org/10.3233/JAD-2008-15110

Ballard, C., Gauthier, S., Corbett, A., Brayne, C., Aarsland, D., & Jones, E. (2011). Alzheimer's disease. *The Lancet*, *377*(9770), 1019–1031. https://doi.org/10.1016/S0140-6736(10)61349-9

Banke, T. G., Bowie, D., Lee, H.-K., Huganir, R. L., Schousboe, A., & Traynelis, S. F. (2000). Control of GluR1 AMPA Receptor Function by cAMP-Dependent Protein Kinase. *The Journal of Neuroscience*, *20*(1), 89–102. https://doi.org/10.1523/JNEUROSCI.20-01-00089.2000

Barnard, N. D., Bush, A. I., Ceccarelli, A., Cooper, J., de Jager, C. A., Erickson, K. I., Fraser, G., Kesler, S., Levin, S. M., Lucey, B., Morris, M. C., & Squitti, R. (2014). Dietary and lifestyle guidelines for the prevention of Alzheimer's disease. *Neurobiology of Aging*, *35*, S74–S78. https://doi.org/10.1016/j.neurobiolaging.2014.03.033

Bostock, E. C. S., Kirkby, K. C., & Taylor, B. V. M. (2017). The Current Status of the Ketogenic Diet in Psychiatry. *Frontiers in Psychiatry*, *8*. https://doi.org/10.3389/fpsyt.2017.00043

Broom, G. M., Shaw, I. C., & Rucklidge, J. J. (2019). The ketogenic diet as a potential treatment and prevention strategy for Alzheimer's disease. *Nutrition*, *60*, 118–121. https://doi.org/10.1016/j.nut.2018.10.003

Butterfield, D. A., & Lauderback, C. M. (2002). Lipid peroxidation and protein oxidation in Alzheimer's disease brain: potential causes and consequences involving amyloid β-peptide-associated free radical oxidative stress 1,2 1Guest Editors: Mark A. Smith and George Perry 2This article is part of a series of reviews on "Causes and Consequences of Oxidative Stress in Alzheimer's Disease." The full list of papers may be found on the homepage of the journal. *Free Radical Biology and Medicine*, *32*(11), 1050–1060. https://doi.org/10.1016/S0891-5849(02)00794-3

Cahill, G. F. (2006). Fuel Metabolism in Starvation. *Annual Review of Nutrition*, *26*(1), 1–22. https://doi.org/10.1146/annurev.nutr.26.061505.111258

Caldeira, C., Oliveira, A. F., Cunha, C., Vaz, A. R., FalcÃ£o, A. S., Fernandes, A., & Brites, D. (2014). Microglia change from a reactive to an age-like phenotype with the time in culture. *Frontiers in Cellular Neuroscience*, *8*. https://doi.org/10.3389/fncel.2014.00152

Campion, D., Dumanchin, C., Hannequin, D., Dubois, B., Belliard, S., Puel, M., Thomas-Anterion, C., Michon, A., Martin, C., Charbonnier, F., Raux, G., Camuzat, A., Penet, C., Mesnage, V., Martinez, M., Clerget-Darpoux, F., Brice, A., & Frebourg, T. (1999). Early-Onset Autosomal Dominant Alzheimer Disease: Prevalence, Genetic Heterogeneity, and Mutation Spectrum. *The American Journal of Human Genetics*, *65*(3), 664–670. https://doi.org/10.1086/302553

Carter, M. D., Simms, G. A., & Weaver, D. F. (2010). The Development of New Therapeutics for Alzheimer's Disease. *Clinical Pharmacology & Therapeutics*, *88*(4), 475–486. https://doi.org/10.1038/clpt.2010.165

Chorley, B. N., Campbell, M. R., Wang, X., Karaca, M., Sambandan, D., Bangura, F., Xue, P., Pi, J., Kleeberger, S. R., & Bell, D. A. (2012). Identification of novel NRF2-regulated genes by ChIP-Seq: influence on retinoid X receptor alpha. *Nucleic Acids Research*, *40*(15), 7416–7429. https://doi.org/10.1093/nar/gks409

Corder, E. H., Saunders, A. M., Strittmatter, W. J., Schmechel, D. E., Gaskell, P. C., Small, G. W., Roses, A. D., Haines, J. L., & Pericak-Vance, M. A. (1993). Gene Dose of Apolipoprotein E Type 4 Allele and the Risk of Alzheimer's Disease in Late Onset Families. *Science*, *261*(5123), 921–923. https://doi.org/10.1126/science.8346443

Dhillon, K. K., & Gupta, S. (2024). *Biochemistry, Ketogenesis*.

Forloni, G., & Balducci, C. (2018). Alzheimer's Disease, Oligomers, and Inflammation. *Journal of Alzheimer's Disease*, *62*(3), 1261–1276. https://doi.org/10.3233/JAD-170819

Fukao, T., Lopaschuk, G. D., & Mitchell, G. A. (2004). Pathways and control of ketone body metabolism: on the fringe of lipid biochemistry. *Prostaglandins, Leukotrienes and Essential Fatty Acids*, *70*(3), 243–251. https://doi.org/10.1016/j.plefa.2003.11.001

Gasior, M., Rogawski, M. A., & Hartman, A. L. (2006). Neuroprotective and disease-modifying effects of the ketogenic diet. *Behavioural Pharmacology*, *17*(5–6), 431–439. https://doi.org/10.1097/00008877-200609000-00009

Goate, A., Chartier-Harlin, M.-C., Mullan, M., Brown, J., Crawford, F., Fidani, L., Giuffra, L., Haynes, A., Irving, N., James, L., Mant, R., Newton, P., Rooke, K., Roques, P., Talbot, C., Pericak-Vance, M., Roses, A., Williamson, R., Rossor, M., … Hardy, J. (1991). Segregation of a missense mutation in the amyloid precursor protein gene with familial Alzheimer's disease. *Nature*, *349*(6311), 704–706. https://doi.org/10.1038/349704a0

Hansen, D. V., Hanson, J. E., & Sheng, M. (2018). Microglia in Alzheimer's disease. *Journal of Cell Biology*, *217*(2), 459–472. https://doi.org/10.1083/jcb.201709069

Harper, M. -E., Bevilacqua, L., Hagopian, K., Weindruch, R., & Ramsey, J. J. (2004). Ageing, oxidative stress, and mitochondrial uncoupling. *Acta Physiologica Scandinavica*, *182*(4), 321–331. https://doi.org/10.1111/j.1365-201X.2004.01370.x

Henderson, S. T., Vogel, J. L., Barr, L. J., Garvin, F., Jones, J. J., & Costantini, L. C. (2009). Study of the ketogenic agent AC-1202 in mild to moderate Alzheimer's disease: a randomized, double-blind, placebo-controlled, multicenter trial. *Nutrition & Metabolism*, *6*(1), 31. https://doi.org/10.1186/1743-7075-6-31

Holmes, C. (2013). Review: Systemic inflammation and <scp>A</scp> lzheimer's disease. *Neuropathology and Applied Neurobiology*, *39*(1), 51–68. https://doi.org/10.1111/j.1365-2990.2012.01301.x

Hughes, S. D., Kanabus, M., Anderson, G., Hargreaves, I. P., Rutherford, T., Donnell, M. O., Cross, J. H., Rahman, S., Eaton, S., & Heales, S. J. R. (2014). The ketogenic diet component decanoic acid increases mitochondrial citrate synthase and complex I activity in neuronal cells. *Journal of Neurochemistry*, *129*(3), 426–433. https://doi.org/10.1111/jnc.12646

Huttenlocher, P. R. (1976). Ketonemia and Seizures: Metabolic and Anticonvulsant Effects of Two Ketogenic Diets in Childhood Epilepsy. *Pediatric Research*, *10*(5), 536–540. https://doi.org/10.1203/00006450-197605000-00006

Kamboh, M. I. (2004). Molecular Genetics of Late-Onset Alzheimer's Disease. *Annals of Human Genetics*, *68*(4), 381–404. https://doi.org/10.1046/j.1529-8817.2004.00110.x

Kashiwaya, Y., Takeshima, T., Mori, N., Nakashima, K., Clarke, K., & Veech, R. L. (2000). <scp>d</scp> -β-Hydroxybutyrate protects neurons in models of Alzheimer's and

Parkinson's disease. *Proceedings of the National Academy of Sciences*, 97(10), 5440–5444. https://doi.org/10.1073/pnas.97.10.5440

Kawai, Y., Garduño, L., Theodore, M., Yang, J., & Arinze, I. J. (2011). Acetylation-Deacetylation of the Transcription Factor Nrf2 (Nuclear Factor Erythroid 2-related Factor 2) Regulates Its Transcriptional Activity and Nucleocytoplasmic Localization. *Journal of Biological Chemistry*, 286(9), 7629–7640. https://doi.org/10.1074/jbc.M110.208173

Kelley, N., Jeltema, D., Duan, Y., & He, Y. (2019). The NLRP3 Inflammasome: An Overview of Mechanisms of Activation and Regulation. *International Journal of Molecular Sciences*, 20(13). https://doi.org/10.3390/ijms20133328

Kim, D. Y., Simeone, K. A., Simeone, T. A., Pandya, J. D., Wilke, J. C., Ahn, Y., Geddes, J. W., Sullivan, P. G., & Rho, J. M. (2015). Ketone bodies mediate antiseizure effects through mitochondrial permeability transition. *Annals of Neurology*, 78(1), 77–87. https://doi.org/10.1002/ana.24424

Lane, C. A., Hardy, J., & Schott, J. M. (2018). Alzheimer's disease. *European Journal of Neurology*, 25(1), 59–70. https://doi.org/10.1111/ene.13439

Lleó, A., Blesa, R., Queralt, R., Ezquerra, M., Molinuevo, J. L., Peña-Casanova, J., Rojo, A., & Oliva, R. (2002). Frequency of Mutations in the Presenilin and Amyloid Precursor Protein Genes in Early-Onset Alzheimer Disease in Spain. *Archives of Neurology*, 59(11), 1759. https://doi.org/10.1001/archneur.59.11.1759

Maalouf, M., Rho, J. M., & Mattson, M. P. (2009). The neuroprotective properties of calorie restriction, the ketogenic diet, and ketone bodies. *Brain Research Reviews*, 59(2), 293–315. https://doi.org/10.1016/j.brainresrev.2008.09.002

Manoharan, S., Guillemin, G. J., Abiramasundari, R. S., Essa, M. M., Akbar, M., & Akbar, M. D. (2016). The Role of Reactive Oxygen Species in the Pathogenesis of Alzheimer's Disease, Parkinson's Disease, and Huntington's Disease: A Mini Review. *Oxidative Medicine and Cellular Longevity*, 2016, 1–15. https://doi.org/10.1155/2016/8590578

Martin, K., Jackson, C. F., Levy, R. G., & Cooper, P. N. (2016). Ketogenic diet and other dietary treatments for epilepsy. *Cochrane Database of Systematic Reviews*, 1–27. https://doi.org/10.1002/14651858.CD001903.pub3

McDonald, T., & Cervenka, M. (2018). The Expanding Role of Ketogenic Diets in Adult Neurological Disorders. *Brain Sciences*, 8(8), 148. https://doi.org/10.3390/brainsci8080148

Medzhitov, R. (2010). Inflammation 2010: New Adventures of an Old Flame. *Cell*, 140(6), 771–776. https://doi.org/10.1016/j.cell.2010.03.006

Nazem, A., Sankowski, R., Bacher, M., & Al-Abed, Y. (2015). Rodent models of neuroinflammation for Alzheimer's disease. *Journal of Neuroinflammation*, 12(1), 74. https://doi.org/10.1186/s12974-015-0291-y

Nolte, R. T., Wisely, G. B., Westin, S., Cobb, J. E., Lambert, M. H., Kurokawa, R., Rosenfeld, M. G., Willson, T. M., Glass, C. K., & Milburn, M. V. (1998). Ligand binding and co-activator assembly of the peroxisome proliferator-activated receptor-γ. *Nature*, 395(6698), 137–143. https://doi.org/10.1038/25931

O'Brien, R. J., & Wong, P. C. (2011). Amyloid Precursor Protein Processing and Alzheimer's Disease. *Annual Review of Neuroscience*, *34*(1), 185–204. https://doi.org/10.1146/annurev-neuro-061010-113613

Offermanns, S. (2017). Hydroxy-Carboxylic Acid Receptor Actions in Metabolism. *Trends in Endocrinology & Metabolism*, *28*(3), 227–236. https://doi.org/10.1016/j.tem.2016.11.007

Palmer, A. M., & Burns, M. A. (1994). Selective increase in lipid peroxidation in the inferior temporal cortex in Alzheimer's disease. *Brain Research*, *645*(1–2), 338–342. https://doi.org/10.1016/0006-8993(94)91670-5

Paoli, A., Bianco, A., Damiani, E., & Bosco, G. (2014). Ketogenic Diet in Neuromuscular and Neurodegenerative Diseases. *BioMed Research International*, *2014*, 1–10. https://doi.org/10.1155/2014/474296

Pinto, A., Bonucci, A., Maggi, E., Corsi, M., & Businaro, R. (2018). Anti-Oxidant and Anti-Inflammatory Activity of Ketogenic Diet: New Perspectives for Neuroprotection in Alzheimer's Disease. *Antioxidants*, *7*(5), 63. https://doi.org/10.3390/antiox7050063

Reger, M. A., Henderson, S. T., Hale, C., Cholerton, B., Baker, L. D., Watson, G. S., Hyde, K., Chapman, D., & Craft, S. (2004). Effects of β-hydroxybutyrate on cognition in memory-impaired adults. *Neurobiology of Aging*, *25*(3), 311–314. https://doi.org/10.1016/S0197-4580(03)00087-3

Reiss, A. B., Arain, H. A., Stecker, M. M., Siegart, N. M., & Kasselman, L. J. (2018). Amyloid toxicity in Alzheimer's disease. *Reviews in the Neurosciences*, *29*(6), 613–627. https://doi.org/10.1515/revneuro-2017-0063

Rusek, M., Pluta, R., Ułamek-Kozioł, M., & Czuczwar, S. J. (2019). Ketogenic Diet in Alzheimer's Disease. *International Journal of Molecular Sciences*, *20*(16), 3892. https://doi.org/10.3390/ijms20163892

Selkoe, D. J. (2001). Alzheimer's Disease: Genes, Proteins, and Therapy. *Physiological Reviews*, *81*(2), 741–766. https://doi.org/10.1152/physrev.2001.81.2.741

Studzinski, C. M., MacKay, W. A., Beckett, T. L., Henderson, S. T., Murphy, M. P., Sullivan, P. G., & Burnham, W. M. (2008). Induction of ketosis may improve mitochondrial function and decrease steady-state amyloid-β precursor protein (APP) levels in the aged dog. *Brain Research*, *1226*, 209–217. https://doi.org/10.1016/j.brainres.2008.06.005

Sullivan, P. G., Rippy, N. A., Dorenbos, K., Concepcion, R. C., Agarwal, A. K., & Rho, J. M. (2004). The ketogenic diet increases mitochondrial uncoupling protein levels and activity. *Annals of Neurology*, *55*(4), 576–580. https://doi.org/10.1002/ana.20062

Swerdlow, R. H. (2011). Brain aging, Alzheimer's disease, and mitochondria. *Biochimica et Biophysica Acta (BBA) - Molecular Basis of Disease*, *1812*(12), 1630–1639. https://doi.org/10.1016/j.bbadis.2011.08.012

Takahashi, R. H., Nagao, T., & Gouras, G. K. (2017). Plaque formation and the intraneuronal accumulation of β-amyloid in Alzheimer's disease. *Pathology International*, *67*(4), 185–193. https://doi.org/10.1111/pin.12520

Tang, Y., & Le, W. (2016). Differential Roles of M1 and M2 Microglia in Neurodegenerative Diseases. *Molecular Neurobiology*, *53*(2), 1181–1194. https://doi.org/10.1007/s12035-014-9070-5

Tanzi, R. E., & Bertram, L. (2005). Twenty Years of the Alzheimer's Disease Amyloid Hypothesis: A Genetic Perspective. *Cell*, *120*(4), 545–555. https://doi.org/10.1016/j.cell.2005.02.008

Van der Auwera, I., Wera, S., Van Leuven, F., & Henderson, S. T. (2005). A ketogenic diet reduces amyloid beta 40 and 42 in a mouse model of Alzheimer's disease. *Nutrition & Metabolism*, *2*(1), 28. https://doi.org/10.1186/1743-7075-2-28

Veech, R. L. (2004). The therapeutic implications of ketone bodies: the effects of ketone bodies in pathological conditions: ketosis, ketogenic diet, redox states, insulin resistance, and mitochondrial metabolism. *Prostaglandins, Leukotrienes and Essential Fatty Acids*, *70*(3), 309–319. https://doi.org/10.1016/j.plefa.2003.09.007

Verdile, G., Keane, K. N., Cruzat, V. F., Medic, S., Sabale, M., Rowles, J., Wijesekara, N., Martins, R. N., Fraser, P. E., & Newsholme, P. (2015). Inflammation and Oxidative Stress: The Molecular Connectivity between Insulin Resistance, Obesity, and Alzheimer's Disease. *Mediators of Inflammation*, *2015*, 1–17. https://doi.org/10.1155/2015/105828

Villemagne, V. L., Burnham, S., Bourgeat, P., Brown, B., Ellis, K. A., Salvado, O., Szoeke, C., Macaulay, S. L., Martins, R., Maruff, P., Ames, D., Rowe, C. C., & Masters, C. L. (2013). Amyloid β deposition, neurodegeneration, and cognitive decline in sporadic Alzheimer's disease: a prospective cohort study. *The Lancet Neurology*, *12*(4), 357–367. https://doi.org/10.1016/S1474-4422(13)70044-9

Vinciguerra, F., Graziano, M., Hagnäs, M., Frittitta, L., & Tumminia, A. (2020). Influence of the Mediterranean and Ketogenic Diets on Cognitive Status and Decline: A Narrative Review. *Nutrients*, *12*(4), 1019. https://doi.org/10.3390/nu12041019

Wang, D., Govindaiah, G., Liu, R., De Arcangelis, V., Cox, C. L., & Xiang, Y. K. (2010). Binding of amyloid β peptide to β 2 adrenergic receptor induces PKA-dependent AMPA receptor hyperactivity. *The FASEB Journal*, *24*(9), 3511–3521. https://doi.org/10.1096/fj.10-156661

Wilkins, H. M., & Swerdlow, R. H. (2017). Amyloid precursor protein processing and bioenergetics. *Brain Research Bulletin*, *133*, 71–79. https://doi.org/10.1016/j.brainresbull.2016.08.009

Winkler, E. A., Nishida, Y., Sagare, A. P., Rege, S. V, Bell, R. D., Perlmutter, D., Sengillo, J. D., Hillman, S., Kong, P., Nelson, A. R., Sullivan, J. S., Zhao, Z., Meiselman, H. J., Wenby, R. B., Soto, J., Abel, E. D., Makshanoff, J., Zuniga, E., De Vivo, D. C., & Zlokovic, B. V. (2015). GLUT1 reductions exacerbate Alzheimer's disease vasculo-neuronal dysfunction and degeneration. *Nature Neuroscience*, *18*(4), 521–530. https://doi.org/10.1038/nn.3966

Włodarek, D. (2019). Role of Ketogenic Diets in Neurodegenerative Diseases (Alzheimer's Disease and Parkinson's Disease). *Nutrients*, *11*(1), 169. https://doi.org/10.3390/nu11010169

Yang, Q., & Zhou, J. (2019). Neuroinflammation in the central nervous system: Symphony of glial cells. *Glia*, *67*(6), 1017–1035. https://doi.org/10.1002/glia.23571

Chapter 4

The Ketogenic Diet in Neuropsychiatric Disorders

Tarsila Elizabeth Juárez-Zepeda[1]
Carmen Rubio[2,*]
Diana Molina-Valdespino[3]
Luis Antonio Marín-Castañeda[2,4]
America Vanoye Carlo[1]
and Leticia Granados-Rojas[1,†]

[1]Laboratorio de Neurociencias II, Instituto Nacional de Pediatría, Mexico City, Mexico
[2]Departamento de Neurofisiología, Instituto Nacional de Neurología y Neurocirugía, Manuel Velasco Suárez, Mexico City, Mexico
[3]Servicio de Salud Mental, Instituto Nacional de Pediatría, Mexico City, Mexico
[4]Facultad Mexicana de Medicina, Universidad La Salle, Mexico City, Mexico

Abstract

The ketogenic diet (KD) is a high fat diet that contains an adequate amount of protein and very low amount of carbohydrates. KD is a perfect strategy to induce a model of biochemical fasting, making the cells to be less dependent on glucose energy substrate and more dependent on ketone bodies to provide the energy need of the body. This switch keeps the body in a state of ketosis, that is, a condition where most of the energy need of the body is obtained from fats. KD was introduced in the 1920s as an effective non-pharmacological treatment for refractory epilepsy. However, in recent years, it was demonstrated to be efficacious in

---

[*] Corresponding Author's Email: macaru4@yahoo.com.mx.
[†] Corresponding Author's Email: lgranados_2000@yahoo.com.mx.

In: The Ketogenic Diet Reexamined
Editors: Leticia Granados-Rojas and Carmen Rubio
ISBN: 979-8-89113-543-7
© 2024 Nova Science Publishers, Inc.

treating neuropsychiatric disorders, such as schizophrenia, autism spectrum disorder, depression, generalized anxiety disorder, and bipolar disorder, which are attributed, in part, to neurotransmission dysfunction mediated by gamma-aminobutyric acid (GABA). These disorders will be addressed in this chapter together with the abnormalities in different components of the GABAergic system, such as the limiting enzyme glutamic acid decarboxylase (GAD), GABA receptors, receptor subunits, isoforms, transporters, as well as neuronal density and GABA levels in each of the psychiatric disorder. In addition, in these neuropsychiatric disorders, the benefits of KD are examined in both clinical studies and animal models. In the same manner, KD action mechanisms to increase GABA synthesis and levels, and to modify different components of the GABAergic system are considered.

Keywords: ketogenic diet, schizophrenia, autism spectrum disorder, depression, generalized anxiety disorder, bipolar disorder, GABA

Acronyms

ACC	Anterior cingulate cortex
ADOS-2	Autism diagnostic observation schedule, 2nd edition
ASD	Autism spectrum disorder
ATEC	Autism treatment evaluation test
BGT-1	Betaine gamma-aminobutyric acid transporter type 1
Ca^{2+}	Calcium
CARS	Childhood autism rating scale
Cl^-	Chloride
DLPFC	Dorsolateral prefrontal cortex
FC	Frontal cortex
GABA	Gamma-aminobutyric acid
$GABA_A$	Gamma-aminobutyric acid receptor type A
$GABA_A$ α	Gamma-aminobutyric acid receptor type A, subunit α
$GABA_A$ α1	Gamma-aminobutyric acid receptor type A, subunit α, isoform 1
$GABA_A$ α2	Gamma-aminobutyric acid receptor type A, subunit α, isoform 2
$GABA_A$ α3	Gamma-aminobutyric acid receptor type A, subunit α, isoform 3

GABA$_A$ α4	Gamma-aminobutyric acid receptor type A, subunit α, isoform 4
GABA$_A$ α5	Gamma-aminobutyric acid receptor type A, subunit α, isoform 5
GABA$_A$ α6	Gamma-aminobutyric acid receptor type A, subunit α, isoform 6
GABA$_A$ β	Gamma-aminobutyric acid receptor type A, subunit β
GABA$_A$ β1	Gamma-aminobutyric acid receptor type A, subunit β, isoform 1
GABA$_A$ β2	Gamma-aminobutyric acid receptor type A, subunit β, isoform 2
GABA$_A$ β3	Gamma-aminobutyric acid receptor type A, subunit β, isoform 3
GABA$_A$ γ	Gamma-aminobutyric acid receptor type A, subunit γ
GABA$_A$ γ1	Gamma-aminobutyric acid receptor type A, subunit γ, isoform 1
GABA$_A$ γ2	Gamma-aminobutyric acid receptor type A, subunit γ, isoform 2
GABA$_A$ γ3	Gamma-aminobutyric acid receptor type A, subunit γ, isoform 3
GABA$_A$ δ	Gamma-aminobutyric acid receptor type A, subunit δ
GABA$_A$ ε	Gamma-aminobutyric acid receptor type A, subunit ε
GABA$_A$ θ	Gamma-aminobutyric acid receptor type A, subunit θ
GABA$_A$ π	Gamma-aminobutyric acid receptor type A, subunit π
GABA$_B$	Gamma-aminobutyric acid receptor type B
GABABR1	Gamma-aminobutyric acid receptor type B, subtype 1
GABABR1a	Gamma-aminobutyric acid receptor type B, subtype 1, isoform a
GABABR1b	Gamma-aminobutyric acid receptor type B, subtype 1, isoform b
GABABR2	Gamma-aminobutyric acid receptor type B, subtype 2
GABA$_C$	Gamma-aminobutyric acid receptor type C
GABA-T	4-aminobutyrate aminotransferase enzyme
GAD	Glutamic acid decarboxylase enzyme
GAD65	Glutamic acid decarboxylase enzyme isotype 65
GAD67	Glutamic acid decarboxylase enzyme isotype 67
GAT	Gamma-aminobutyric acid transporter
GAT-1	Gamma-aminobutyric acid transporter type 1
GAT-2	Gamma-aminobutyric acid transporter type 2

GAT-3	Gamma-aminobutyric acid transporter type 3
KCC2	K^+/Cl^- cation-chloride cotransporter 2
KD	Ketogenic diet
MCT	Medium-chain triglycerides
MK-801	Dizocilpine
mRNA	Messenger RNA
MRS	Magnetic resonance spectroscopy
PANSS	Positive and negative symptom scale
PFC	Prefrontal cortex
PV	Parvalbumin
SSA	Succinic semialdehyde
VGAT	Vesicular gamma-aminobutyric acid transporter
VPA	Valproic acid

Introduction

Ketogenic Diet

Ketogenic diet (KD) is characterized by high fat, low carbohydrate, and moderate protein intake that switch the body into a metabolic state known as ketosis, where the body utilizes ketone bodies for energy. The classic KD maintains a 4:1 macronutrient ratio, i.e., four grams of fat for every gram of carbohydrate and protein combined, thereby primarily making the body toderive its calorie needs from fats (McDonald & Cervenka, 2018). KD acts as a metabolic simulation of fasting, initiating ketone body synthesis once the liver's glycogen stores are exhausted (Fedorovich et al., 2018).

First introduced in the 1920s, KD has gained recognition as a non-pharmaceutical intervention for refractory epilepsy with promising outcomes (Höhn et al., 2019). However, the advent of diphenylhydantoin in 1938 led to a progressive decline in the popularity of KD (Wheless, 2008).

Despite this, recent research has re-established the efficacy of KD in managing a spectrum of neurological conditions including traumatic brain injury (McDougall et al., 2018); ischemia (Shaafi et al., 2014); and several neuropsychiatric disorders, such as schizophrenia (Sarnyai et al., 2019), autism spectrum disorder (Napoli et al., 2014), depression (Ricci et al., 2020), anxiety (Włodarczyk et al., 2020), and bipolar disorder (Campbell and Campbell, 2020).

Dysfunction in gamma-aminobutyric acid (GABA)-mediated neurotransmission is implicated in numerous neuropsychiatric disorders. In recent times, evidence from both clinical trials and animal studies has demonstrated KD´s potential in treating disorders attributed, in part, to disruptions in GABA-mediated neurotransmission.

GABAergic System

GABA is known to be the dominant inhibitory neurotransmitter in adult mammalian nervous system. This neurotransmitter is synthesized when glutamate is decarboxylated by glutamic acid decarboxylase (GAD) enzyme, which is commonly found in two isotypes: GAD65 and GAD67. Following its synthesis, GABA is packaged into synaptic vesicles by the vesicular GABA transporter (VGAT). The release of GABA into the synaptic cleft by GABAergic interneurons is triggered by a Ca^{2+}-mediated fusion of the vesicle membrane with the presynaptic neuron membrane, an event made possible by presynaptic action potential. GABA operates through three receptor types: $GABA_A$, $GABA_B$, and $GABA_C$. The ionotropic receptors, which are $GABA_A$ and $GABA_C$, are ligand-gated chloride (Cl^-) channels that, upon GABA's binding, facilitate the influx of Cl^- into the neuron and thus, bring about membrane hyperpolarization and a reduction in neuronal excitability. $GABA_A$ receptors, which are heteropentameric protein complexes located on the postsynaptic membrane of inhibitory neurons, mediate fast neuronal inhibition in milliseconds and produce most of the physiological actions of GABA. These receptors are characterized by several subunits: α, β, γ, δ, ε, π, and θ, some of which have multiple isoforms represented as α1-6, β1-3, and γ1-3. $GABA_B$ receptor is available in two subtypes — GABABR1 and GABABR2. GABABR1 subunit occurs in two isoforms: GABABR1a and GABABR1b. It is a metabotropic type receptor and regulates slow-inhibitory response. GABAc receptor is composed of multiple subunits of the same subtype and can be either ρ1 or ρ2. The termination of the action of GABA is facilitated by its uptake into neurons and glia through GABA transporters (GAT) located in the cellular membranes. These transporters are classified into GAT-1, GAT-2, GAT-3, and BGT-1. GAT-1 is the most prevalent in the brain and is primarily responsible for GABA reuptake. Once internalized, GABA can either be repackaged into vesicles or be metabolized to succinic semialdehyde (SSA) by the enzyme 4-aminobutyrate aminotransferase (GABA-T). The latter is crucial for the metabolic inactivation of GABA. SSA is subsequently converted to succinate, which enters the tricarboxylic acid cycle and is eventually transformed back into glutamate (Pizzarelli & Cherubini, 2011; Cherubini, 2012; Rogawski et al., 2016; Di et al., 2020).

Given that GABA plays a pivotal role in the assembly and formation of neuronal circuits in developing brain, the dysfunction of GABA-mediated neurotransmission has been associated with various neuropsychiatric disorders (Cellot & Cherubini, 2014), including schizophrenia, autism spectrum disorder, depression, generalized anxiety disorder, and bipolar disorder.

Ketogenic Diet and GABAergic System

The underlying mechanism through which KD exerts its effects remains largely unclear. It has been proposed that the therapeutic benefits of KD in the treatment of neurological and neuropsychiatric conditions derive from alterations in various components and metabolic processes of the GABAergic system. Thus, Yudkoff et al. (2005), postulated that increased synthesis or levels of the inhibitory neurotransmitter GABA could elucidate the activities of KD that resulted in harnessing its therapeutic benefits. It was thought that the underlying event resides in a mechanism that reduces the conversion of glutamate to aspartate; thus, leaving more glutamate available for GABA synthesis.

Though studies in animal models have yielded inconsistent outcomes, research has indicated a correlation between increased ketone bodies and elevated GABA levels in synaptosomes (Erecińska et al., 1996). A study conducted by Calderón et al. (2017) using *in vivo* microdialysis in rats subjected to a 15-day KD regime also reported augmented GABA levels in the rat hippocampus, suggesting potential benefits for disorders characterized by GABA deficiency. However, Yudkoff et al. (2001) reported a decline in GABA levels in the mouse cerebellum after a three-day KD treatment, with no observed changes in the forebrain of the mice. In line with this finding are the reports of some authors who did not find any significant alterations in GABA levels in various brain regions of rats and mice following KD treatment (Appleton & DeVivo, 1974; Melø et al., 2006; Gzielo et al., 2020; Al-Mudallal et al., 1996; Yudkoff et al., 2005).

Interestingly, different from animal models, human studies have demonstrated an increase in GABA levels. Magnetic resonance spectroscopy (MRS) research by Wang et al. (2003) revealed elevated GABA levels in two out of four patients. Similar findings were reported by Dahlin et al. (2005) who indicated an increased GABA levels in the cerebrospinal fluid of children with refractory epilepsy following KD treatment.

A 7-day KD administration, with moderate caloric restriction, elevated the expressions of GAD65 and GAD67 by messenger RNA (mRNA) in rats. The isoform GAD65 was expressed in the inferior and superior colliculi and cerebellar cortex, while the isoform GAD67 was expressed in the superior colliculus, temporal cortex, and striatum. This suggests the influence of KD in GABA synthesis (Cheng et al., 2004). In the hippocampus, no notable impact of KD on GAD67 was found (Lauritzen et al., 2016).

In relation to $GABA_A$ receptor subunits, research conducted by Lauritzen et al. (2016) indicated that in the mouse hippocampus, KD augmented the expression of the α1 subunit without any effect on the γ2 subunit.

β-hydroxybutyrate, a ketone body synthesized during KD treatment, diminished GABA-T mRNA expression in cultured astrocytes. This event implies a potential increase in GABA levels by inhibiting its degradation (Suzuki et al., 2009).

Lastly, a study by Granados-Rojas et al. (2020) showed that the administration of KD during three months brings about an increased expression of K^+/Cl^- cation-chloride cotransporter 2 (KCC2) in the rat dentate gyrus. KCC2 plays a crucial role in modulating the concentration of intracellular Cl^- within neurons, which determines the strength and polarity of GABA-mediated neurotransmission.

Neuropsychiatric Disorders

The Ketogenic Diet in Schizophrenia

Schizophrenia is a complex heterogenous, multifactorial and chronic psychiatric disorder, primarily associated with elevated dopamine release and an increase in D2 receptors (Seeman and Kapur, 2000). In the same way, Sigvard et al. (2023) found that GABA and glutamate neurotransmitter systems are involved in the development of psychosis.

The clinical manifestations of schizophrenia encompass a diverse array of symptoms, which can be grouped into positive and negative. The positive symptoms consist of hallucinations, delusions, disorganized thoughts or speech, and peculiar behaviors while the negatives include all those characterized by lack of motivation, drive, enjoyment, and social interactions. In addition, it is a disorder that is also marked by cognitive dysfunction, impacting on attention, memory, executive functioning, and social interactions, as well as on motor disturbances (Kahn et al., 2015; Maroney, 2020).

Schizophrenia and GABA

Numerous studies suggest metabolic alterations and variations in the components of the GABAergic system in individuals with schizophrenia. Evidence from post-mortem studies on subjects with schizophrenia reveals a decline in the expression of GAD67 mRNA and protein, particularly in the prefrontal cortex (PFC) (Guidotti et al., 2000; Curley et al., 2011). This reduced expression also extends to other cortical regions, including the orbitofrontal and superior temporal cortices, as well as the striatum and thalamus (Thompson et al., 2009).

A significant decrease in GAD65 has been identified in the primary auditory cortex of individuals diagnosed with schizophrenia (Moyer et al., 2012). However, existing research has not reported any alterations in the expression of GAD65 in the PFC in patients suffering from schizophrenia (Glausier et al., 2015).

Furthermore, in schizophrenic patients, a notable reduction in the levels of GAT-1 mRNA has been reported in various regions of the brain, including the PFC (Ohnuma et al., 1999; Volk et al., 2001), dorsolateral prefrontal cortex (DLPFC) (Hashimoto et al., 2008a, b), anterior cingulate cortex (ACC) and both visual and motor cortices (Hashimoto et al., 2008a). Additional studies have indicated an increased binding of postsynaptic $GABA_A$ receptors in several brain regions, such as PFC (Benes et al., 1996a), DLPFC (Dean et al., 1999), ACC (Benes et al., 1992), and the hippocampal formation (Benes et al., 1996b).

Extensive studies that were focused on different subunits of $GABA_A$ receptor in the PFC of schizophrenic patients yielded varied results. An increase in $GABA_A$ receptor α1 subunit mRNA and protein was documented in the PFC of these patients in studies performed by Impagnatiello et al. (1998), Ohnuma et al. (1999), and Ishikawa et al. (2004). However, in the studies of Hashimoto et al. (2008a, b) and Beneyto et al. (2011), contrasting findings in the DLPFC were reported. Nevertheless, in the studies of Akbarian et al. (1995) and Duncan et al. (2010), no changes were found in PFC and DLPFC respectively. In the cases of α2 and α3 subunits, an increase in $GABA_A$ receptor α2 subunit mRNA in DLPFC and protein in PFC was observed (Volk et al., 2002), while the α3 subunit mRNA did not exhibit any change in DLPFC (Beneyto et al., 2011).

Divergent results were noted for the α4 and α5 subunits. The α4 subunit mRNA showed a reduction in PFC (Hashimoto et al., 2008b; Maldonado-Avilés et al., 2009), whereas the α5 subunit mRNA increased in PFC according to Impagnatiello et al. (1998). However, several studies have indicated a reduction in DLPFC (Duncan et al., 2010; Beneyto et al., 2011), and others reported no change in PFC for the α5 subunit (Akbarian et al., 1995). Studies on β-type subunits also revealed mixed results. Beneyto et al. (2011) reported no alterations in GABA$_A$ receptor β1 mRNA in DLPFC. For the β2 subunit, both an increase in PFC (Ishikawa et al., 2004) and a decrease have been observed (Beneyto et al., 2011). The β3 subunit levels were increased in the PFC (Ishikawa et al., 2004), but other studies showed a reduction (Hashimoto et al., 2008b), and some found no changes (Beneyto et al., 2011).

Regarding the γ2 and δ subunits, two studies reported a reduction in GABA$_A$ γ2 mRNA in the DLPFC (Huntsman et al., 1998; Hashimoto et al., 2008b), while another study found no alterations in the PFC (Akbarian et al., 1995). In addition, a reduction was observed in GABA$_A$ receptor δ subunit mRNA (Hashimoto et al., 2008b; Maldonado-Avilés et al., 2009).

As for GABA$_B$ receptors, Fatemi et al. (2011) showed reductions in protein levels of the two GABA$_B$ receptor subunits GABABR1 and GABABR2 in lateral cerebellum. Ishikawa et al. (2005) also indicated a reduction of the GABABR1a protein in PFC.

GABAergic interneurons are the principal inhibitory neurons. Several studies performed on post-mortem brain tissue of patients with schizophrenia have reported alterations in neuronal density. Whereas most of these studies showed decreased cell densities in various brain regions such as frontal cortex (FC) (Benes et al., 1991), the cingulate cortex (Benes, 1991), the entorhinal cortex (Wang et al., 2011) and the hippocampus (Konradi et al., 2011), others reported an increase, for instance, in the FC (Joshi et al., 2012). Schizophrenic patients showed a deficit in the density of parvalbumin (PV)-immunoreactive interneurons in the hippocampus (Zhang & Reynolds, 2002).

Decreased levels of GAD67 and GAT-1, in addition to increased expression of the GABA$_A$ receptor subunits in post-mortem studies mentioned above, suggest a decrease in GABA production in schizophrenia. In this line, the neuroimaging studies of GABA levels using MRS help in finding *in vivo* evidence in specific regions; however, such imaging studies have yielded variable results in patients with schizophrenia. Thus, decreased levels of

GABA have been reported in ACC (Rowland et al., 2013), PFC (Marsman et al., 2014), and basal ganglia (Goto et al., 2010), while other studies have reported increased GABA levels (Kegeles et al., 2012) in the medial PFC cortex, or have shown no changes in DLPFC (Kegeles et al., 2012), in the frontal lobe (Goto et al., 2010), ACC (Brandt et al., 2016) and PFC (Chen et al., 2017).

These varied findings underline the complexity of schizophrenia and indicate that alterations in GABAergic interneurons and GABA levels are region-specific, contributing to the multifaceted nature of this psychiatric disorder. The discrepancies observed across different studies suggest that further research is essential to unravel the intricate relationship between GABAergic system alterations and schizophrenia.

Ketogenic Diet Research in Schizophrenia

Since 1965, there have been instances demonstrating the potential beneficial effects of KD in patients with chronic schizophrenia. One of the earliest studies carried out in ten female patients showed a notable decrease (Beckomberga Rating Scale) in symptoms after two weeks on KD. However, it is worth noting that this study was small and poorly controlled, and this could limit the generalizability of the findings. Interestingly, when KD was discontinued, an increase in symptomatology was observed, albeit the symptoms were better than the initial rating (Pacheco et al., 1965). Moreover, there are several case reports that have highlighted the potential benefits of KD in managing schizophrenia. One such report was a 70-year-old woman diagnosed with schizophrenia and who did not experience auditory or visual hallucinations after 12 months on KD (Kraft & Westman, 2009).

Another report by Palmer et al., (2017) described two cases of individuals with schizoaffective disorder. Both patients, in response to KD treatment, experienced significant reductions in their positive and negative symptoms, measured by the Positive and Negative Symptom Scale (PANSS). However, the symptoms of the patients, just as reported in other studies, returned when KD was discontinued and improved again when it was resumed.

The findings of studies of Palmer et al. (2019) and Gilbert-Jaramillo et al. (2018) contributed to the growing body of evidence, which showed KD as having therapeutic potential for individuals with schizophrenia. In the study by Palmer et al. (2019), two female patients with a long history of schizophrenia and psychotic symptoms experienced complete remission of their symptoms without the need for antipsychotic medications after several years on KD. These cases are particularly noteworthy given the chronic nature of the patient's symptoms and their ability to achieve remission and functional restoration through the diet. Similarly, the study by Gilbert-Jaramillo et al. (2018) involving 22-year-old opposite-sex twin with schizophrenia showed promising results. Both patients experienced an improvement in psychiatric symptoms after approximately 14 consecutive days of moderate/high ketosis on a 3:1 ratio KD. Additionally, there was a noticeable trend of decreasing PANSS scores during ketosis, further supporting the potential benefits of KD in ameliorating psychiatric symptoms in schizophrenia.

Research using animal models has consistently demonstrated the potential efficacy of KD in addressing schizophrenia. One study conducted by Tregellas et al. (2015) delved into the impact of KD on hippocampal P20/N40 gating in DBA/2 mice, an established endophenotype mirroring the inhibitory deficits observable in P50 sensory gating among individuals with schizophrenia. P50 gating deficits describes a situation where patients are unable to filter the initial neuronal response, occurring 50 ms post-stimulus, to a second stimulus in a pair of identical, repetitive auditory clicks. Notably, those animals exhibiting the highest ketone levels displayed the most reduced P20/N40 gating ratios, thereby suggesting a potential improvement in sensory gating deficits associated with schizophrenia through KD. Furthermore, Kraeuter et al. (2015) provided evidence of KD mitigating pathological behaviors in an N-Methyl-D-aspartate receptor hypo-function model of schizophrenia. This model was induced by an acute injection of dizocilpine (MK-801) in male C57BL/6 mice. KD was found to moderate the effects of low-dose MK-801, leading to a reduction in hyperactivity, stereotyped behavior, and ataxia. Additionally, KD normalized impairments in social interaction and spatial working memory induced by MK801. Building on these findings, Kraeuter et al. (2019) further reported, utilizing the same schizophrenia model, that KD was able to prevent MK-801-induced impairments in prepulse inhibition of startle, a recognized endophenotype of schizophrenia at both the 3 and 7-week.

Nevertheless, despite the promising results depicted in the existing literature, there remains a need for more extensive controlled randomized trials to further validate the benefits of KD in treating schizophrenia (Sarnyai et al., 2019).

The Ketogenic Diet in Autism Spectrum Disorder

Autism Spectrum Disorder (ASD) is a neurodevelopmental disorder that encompasses a variety of early-onset social communication challenges, coupled with the presence of restricted interests and repetitive sensory-motor behaviors. Both genetic predispositions and environmental elements are recognized as contributing factors to the development of ASD (Cellot & Cherubini, 2014; Kerub et al., 2018; Lord et al., 2018; Hodges et al., 2020). It is crucial to highlight the elevated prevalence of epilepsy within the ASD population, marking a significant correlation between the two conditions (Hodges et al., 2020).

Autism Spectrum Disorder and GABA

Past research posits that abnormalities in glutamate and GABAergic circuits play a role in the pathophysiology of ASD (Di et al., 2020). There were reductions in GAD65 and GAD67 in the parietal and cerebellar regions of post-mortem brains from individuals with autism (Yip et al., 2007). Furthermore, diminished density of both $GABA_A$ (Oblak et al., 2009) and $GABA_B$ (Oblak et al., 2010) receptors in the ACC have been documented in post-mortem brain tissues from ASD patients.

Additionally, studies by Fatemi et al. (2009a) revealed decreased expression of four $GABA_A$ receptor subunits α1-3 and β3 in the parietal cortex, while α1 and β3 levels were found to be lower in the cerebellum. Subsequent research by Fatemi et al. (2009b) identified a decrease in $GABA_B$ receptors (GABABR1 and GABABR2) in the cerebellum of post-mortem autistic brains. An unbiased stereological study indicated an upsurge in the expression of GABAergic interneurons, expressing calcium-binding proteins in the hippocampal formation of ASD individuals (Lawrence et al., 2010). Besides, multiple studies employing MRS have reported diminished GABA levels in ASD patients. For instance, Rojas et al. (2014) found reduced GABA levels in the perisylvian region of the left hemisphere, while Puts et al. (2017) proposed that GABA levels are decreased in sensorimotor regions but remain stable in occipital visual areas.

Insights from studies that employed ASD animal models have similarly reported anomalies in GABAergic functions. These anomalies encompassed reduced GABA release in the amygdala (Olmos-Serrano et al., 2010), decreased expression of GAD65 and GAD67 (Chao et al., 2010), decreased expression of $GABA_A$ receptors (Sinkkonen et al., 2003), as well as lower number of PV-immunoreactive interneurons (Kobayashi et al., 2018), and a decreased number of GABAergic interneurons (Chao et al., 2010).

Ketogenic Diet Research in Autism Spectrum

Numerous dietary regimens for individuals with ASD have been the focus of extensive research in recent years. KD has demonstrated promising outcomes for patients with ASD across various clinical studies. However, the exact mechanism underlying the beneficial impact of KD remains uncertain. Several proposed mechanisms have been put forth, including the restoration of metabolic processes. These mechanisms potentially involve the GABAergic and cholinergic systems and are theorized to influence inflammatory pathways, mitochondrial function, oxidative stress, and the gut microbiome (Alam et al., 2023).

Evangeliou et al. (2003) conducted a pilot prospective follow-up study, examining the role of KD in 18 children exhibiting autistic behavior. The diet was administered for six months, comprising four-week intervals of continuous diet followed by two-week diet-free intervals. Improvements in the children were noted in several parameters following the Childhood Autism Rating Scale (CARS). In a separate study by El-Rashidy et al. (2017), 15 aged 3-8 years children diagnosed with ASD were put on Atkins/KD for six months, showcasing improvements on both the Autism Treatment Evaluation Test (ATEC) and CARS scores in comparison to a control group, with notable advancements in cognition and sociability.

Furthermore, Zarnowska et al. (2018), reported unparalleled improvement in a case study of a 6-year-old high-functioning autistic patient with subclinical epileptic discharges and notable glucose hypometabolism in the brain who was treated with KD. A month after initiating the KD, significant enhancements in the patient's behavior and intellectual abilities were observed, including improvements in hyperactivity, attention span, reactions to stimuli, adaptability, communication skills, and emotional responses. These advancements persisted through the 16-month observation period.

Lee et al. (2018) conducted an open-label, observer-blinded clinical trial in a group of 15 children with ASD. The trial aimed to assess the feasibility and efficacy of a modified KD gluten-free diet supplemented with medium-chain triglycerides (MCT) for ameliorating core clinical impairments. Significant improvements were noted in core autism features as assessed by the Autism Diagnostic Observation Schedule, 2nd edition (ADOS-2) after 3 and 6 months on the diet protocol. Moreover, improvements in CARS items related to imitation, body use, and fear or nervousness after three months were noted. This suggested that a modified gluten-free KD with supplemental MCT could potentially be a beneficial treatment option for addressing core features of ASD.

Lastly, Mu et al. (2020) conducted another similar open-label, observer-blinded clinical trial involving 17 children with ASD that explored the benefits of a modified KD gluten-free diet with MCT. The findings revealed a reduction in the overall ADOS-2 score after three months of KD treatment, indicating the potential therapeutic benefits of such dietary modifications.

In ASD animal models, KD has shown promising results. Ahn et al. (2014) studied its effects on mice with autism induced by prenatal exposure to valproic acid (VPA), reporting that KD mitigated the social behavior deficits observed in this ASD model. VPA mice exhibited increased social impairment, repetitive behavior, and a higher nociceptive threshold. Remarkably, those in the VPA group fed with KD displayed improvements in social behavior, with elevated sociability and social novelty index scores compared to VPA mice on a standard diet (Castro et al., 2017). This study suggests that KD can counteract all VPA-induced behaviors, modifying social behaviors and mitochondrial respiration as observed in this ASD model.

The BTBR mouse strain is characterized by low sociability, reduced communication, and elevated self-directed behavior and can serve as another ASD animal model. Ruskin et al. (2013) demonstrated that KD amelioratedautistic behavior in BTBR mice. In addition, Ruskin et al. (2017) studied maternal immune activation in pregnant C57Bl/6 mice as an ASD model, finding that the male offspring exhibited social deficits and high levels of repetitive behavior, which were partially or entirely reversed by KD. Dai et al. (2017) used Glu3+/- mice as another ASD model and discovered that KD notably improved sociability. Additionally, alterations in the Engrailed genes, particularly Engrailed 2, can have neurodevelopmental consequences and result in autism-related behavior. Verpeut et al. (2016) utilized this model to demonstrate that KD exposure led to short-term improvements in social interactions and appropriate exploratory behaviors.

However, despite these promising findings, several aspects, including the role of microbiota, variations in phenotypes, immunological dysfunction, and long-term effects of KD, still require further understanding and exploration.

Ketogenic Diet in Depression

Depression is a prevalent and a notably heterogeneous psychiatric disorder with a diverse etiological spectrum, which encompasses genetic susceptibility, adverse childhood factors, lifestyle choices, psychological stressors, and systemic inflammatory conditions (Luscher & Fuchs, 2015). The syndrome is characterized by enduring symptoms such as pervasive sadness, feelings of hopelessness and helplessness, diminished self-worth, and a loss of interest or pleasure in activities that were once fulfilling or enjoyable (World Health Organization, 2021).

Theories consider psychosocial stress in predisposed individuals, which brings about dysfunction in neurotransmitter circuits, such as serotonin, norepinephrine, dopamine, glutamate and GABA, with a consecutive endocrine response circuits and immune dysfunction (Hasler, 2010).

Depression and GABA

A diminished concentration of GABA in the brain, alongside a modified expression and function of GABA$_A$ receptors and alterations in GABAergic signaling, are implicated in the etiology of major depressive disorder (Möhler, 2012; Luscher & Fuchs, 2015). Initial investigations disclosed reduced levels of GABA in cerebrospinal fluid (Gold et al., 1980). Price et al. (2009) corroborated the reduced presence of GABA in major depressive disorder.

Additional studies on depressed patients have revealed decreased expression of GABA$_A$-benzodiazepine receptor binding in regions such as the parahippocampal temporal gyrus and the right lateral superior temporal gyrus (Klumpers et al., 2010). Analyses in the left DLPFC of depressed suicide victims demonstrated an altered expression of numerous GABA receptor-subunit genes that were primarily upregulated (GABA$_A$ β3, GABA$_A$ δ, and GABA$_A$ γ2), (Choudary et al., 2005). Alterations in the secretion of hormones like oxytocin, cortisol/corticosterone, corticotropin-releasing hormone, and adrenocorticotropic hormone have established connections with depression and anxiety (Kalueff & Nutt, 2007). Additionally, GABA plays a crucial role in inhibiting the release of cortisol and corticotropin-releasing hormone during stress (Włodarczyk et al., 2021).

In some reports of patients with depressive symptoms, KD has shown to have a beneficial effect that may lead to euthymia (Wlodarczyk et al., 2021) similar to that provided by some antidepressants (Stafstrom & Rho, 2012).

Ketogenic Diet Research in Depression

KD has been researched as an alternative or addition to the use of antidepressants, particularly in animal models. There is a growing body of evidence supporting the need for further clinical trials in human patients to validate the efficacy of KD in treating depression. According to Ricci et al. (2020), KD has exhibited promising outcomes, such as reduced oxidative stress, enhanced mitochondrial function, and anti-inflammatory effects. These effects include a reduction in pro-inflammatory cytokine levels, such as TNF-alpha and IL-1, and alterations in the gut microbiota strains, which have been associated with major depressive disorders.

Patients experiencing depression often exhibit alterations in appetite, manifested as either overeating or reduced food intake (hyporexia). Despite these challenges, the incorporation of KD may offer potential benefits. KD can serve dual roles. First, it can act as an appetite stimulant by increasing GABA concentrations in the brain and decreasing reactive oxygen species. Secondly, it can act as an appetite suppressant by reducing the phosphorylation of adenosine monophosphate-activated protein and elevating post-meal free fatty acid levels (Włodarczyk et al., 2020).

Several studies have indicated the potential benefits of KD in managing depressive symptoms. Włodarczyk et al. (2021) highlighted that patients exhibiting depressive symptoms may experience a positive impact, such as euthymic state, when treated with KD, an effect akin to the benefits offered by certain antidepressants (Stafstrom & Rho, 2012).

Likewise, different analyses of animals subjected to KD underscored the prospective use of KD as an alternative treatment for depression. A notable experiment involving a set of 40 adult male Wistar rats, subjected to a 4:1 KD or a control diet for a week and later to the Porsolt Test, revealed significant findings. The results demonstrated that the KD group of rats exhibited less immobility compared to the control group, indicating lower "behavioral despair" in KD rats, similar to those treated with antidepressants (Murphy et al., 2004).

Moreover, another research performed with mice brought to light some intriguing anatomical outcomes. Among these are neuroanatomical alterations marked by a 4.8% increase in cerebellar volume, a 1.39% decrease in hypothalamic volume, and a 4.77% reduction in corpus callosum volume in the brains of mice subjected to prenatal KD exposures. These anatomical changes were associated with behavioral modifications, such as decreased susceptibility to anxiety and depression, and increased tendency towards hyperactivity in adult life compared to the control group (Sussman et al., 2015).

Ketogenic Diet in Generalized Anxiety Disorder

Generalized Anxiety Disorder is characterized by persistent and excessive anxiety or worry occurring on the majority of days for a minimum of six months. This condition is also manifested through symptoms such as restlessness, muscle tension, sleep disturbances, and diminished attention. Individuals with generalized anxiety disorder often experience disruptions in various areas of life, including school, work, social engagements, and daily activities. Notably, there exists a significant comorbidity with major depressive disorders (National Institutes of Health, 2021a; Möhler, 2012).

Anxiety Disorder and GABA

The involvement of GABA in mood disorders has been postulated since 1980 in studies conducted by Emrich et al. (1980). These authors suggested that reduced GABA levels could be associated with mood fluctuations and the manifestation of anxiety. Furthermore, it has been documented that positive allosteric modulators of GABA alleviate anxiety symptoms. The modulation of GABAergic neurotransmission within the amygdala presents a compelling avenue for the management of anxiety-related responses. Specifically, administering GABA or GABA receptor agonists directly into the amygdala has been found to decrease indicators of fear and anxiety (Nuss, 2015). In addition, evidence points to a reduction in the number of $GABA_A$ receptors located in the temporal lobe (Włodarczyk et al., 2020).

A research involving mice has demonstrated that intra-amygdala infusions of GABA-positive allosteric modulator, along with $GABA_A$ receptor antagonist, mitigated anxiety-like behavior, exhibiting a tendency towards anxiolytic effects (Barbalho et al., 2009). Besides, developmental irregularities in GABAergic inhibition within the brain have been associated with behavioral and endocrine anomalies. Specifically, the heterozygous inactivation of the γ2 subunit gene of the $GABA_A$ receptor in mouse embryos has been linked to indicative of trait anxiety (Shen et al., 2010). In the brain, ionotropic type A receptors for GABA are identified as targets for anxiolytic and sedative medications, and hold a vital regulatory function in the locus coeruleus. Many differences have been observed in the expression profiles of the α1 and γ2 subunits in the locus coeruleus across species. Notably, the benzodiazepine sites related to sedation are found to be more significant in humans as compared to rodents (Hellsten et al., 2010).

Ketogenic Diet Research in Anxiety Disorder

The use of KD in controlled studies of generalized anxiety disorders has not shown robust evidence that may help to identify which patients would benefit from KD (Dietch et al., 2023).

Despite the above, some authors have claimed that anxiety is related to depression, with shared symptoms and pathological mechanisms, pointing out the common neuronal dysfunctions in both disorders (Möhler, 2012).

In mice, prenatal exposure to KD results in behavioral alterations, including reduced susceptibility to anxiety (Sussman et al. 2015). In rats, the intake of ketogenic supplements reduces anxiety-related behavior and may exert its alleviating effect on anxiety levels via the GABAergic system (Ari et al., 2016). Studies on GABA receptors reported a limited reduction of $GABA_A$, mainly in the hippocampus and cerebral cortex; showing enhanced behavioral inhibition toward natural aversive stimuli (Crestani et al., 1999). GABABR1 deficiency shows anxiety and panic-like behavior (Möhler, 2012).

The Ketogenic Diet in Bipolar Disorder

Bipolar disorder encompasses various forms, among which are Bipolar I and Bipolar II, each with distinct symptomatology. Bipolar I, is characterized by the presence of, at least, one manic episode, during which individuals may experience elevated mood, a sense of grandiosity, heightened energy and activity levels, significant distractibility, and a rapid flow of ideas, among other symptoms. On the other hand, Bipolar II is marked by the occurrence of a major depressive episode and a hypomanic episode, both of which can significantly impair social and occupational functioning (National Institutes of Health, 2021b).

Bipolar Disorder and GABA

GABAergic dysfunction has been postulated as a contributing factor to affective or mood disorders (Emrich et al., 1980; Brambilla et al., 2003). However, research findings in this area have been somewhat inconsistent. For instance, a study by Kaufman et al. (2009) did not identify significant differences in the levels of GABA, glutamate, or glutamine between patients diagnosed with bipolar disorder and the control group, as assessed through MRS. Contrastingly, another study reported an elevated GABA/creatine ratio in participants with bipolar disorder in comparison to healthy controls (Brady et al., 2013). Additionally, some research has indicated a trend toward a negative correlation between perisylvian GABA levels and scores on the Hamilton Depression Rating Scale (Atagün et al., 2017).

Fatemi et al. (2017) identified four patterns of GABAergic disorders: higher expression of $GABA_A$ receptor α subunits; lower expression of $GABA_A$

receptor β subunits; higher expression of the $GABA_A$ receptor ε subunit, and lower expression of $GABA_B$ receptor subunits. In rat, preclinical studies based on mood stabilizer Lithium, a standard treatment for bipolar disorder (Won & Kim, 2017) that has shown an increase of GABA levels in rat brain (Vargas et al., 1998; Brambilla et al., 2003), showed that the GABAergic system is related to mood disorders. Further research and clinical trials with a more significant number of participants are necessary to confirm the hypothesis and relationship of KD.

Ketogenic Diet Research in Bipolar Disorder
The effects of KD on bipolar disorder are still not fully understood. Nonetheless, existing case reports and studies have provided promising insights, and have prompted the need for more comprehensive research and clinical trials on the topic. For example, a controlled analytic study conducted by Campbell and Campbell (2019) investigated online reports from 274 patients diagnosed with bipolar disorder. The study concluded that the strength of the association and the sustained benefits reported support the hypothesis that KD may have favorable effects on mood stabilization. Additionally, Phelps et al. (2013) documented cases of two women with type II bipolar disorder who maintained ketosis for an extended time and experienced more significant mood stabilization than what was achieved with medication alone.

KD is speculated to mimic the pharmacological impacts of mood stabilizers by restoring mitochondrial function and energy metabolism. However, the biochemical mechanisms underlying the variations in the type of bipolar disorder and the impact of KD on each type remain to be fully elucidated (Yu & Shebani, 2021).

Conclusion

In summary, evidences from post-mortem human reports, clinical research in psychiatric patients, and animal models point out the important role of GABA in the pathophysiology of various psychiatric disorders, such as schizophrenia, autism spectrum disorder, depression, generalized anxiety disorder, and bipolar disorder. KD has shown efficacy in disorders linked with dysfunction of GABA circuits. In addition, evidence indicates that KD positively modifies the GABAergic system. However, for depression, anxiety, and bipolar disorder, there are no conclusive studies on the benefits and drawbacks of KD in these patients. Further research with rigorously controlled studies is needed to elucidate KD action mechanisms and to support with evidence-based medicine, the clinical benefits of various psychiatric disorders where GABA-mediated neurotransmission dysfunction has been hypothesized.

Disclaimer

None.

References

Ahn, Y., Narous, M., Tobias, R., Rho, J. M., & Mychasiuk, R. (2014). The ketogenic diet modifies social and metabolic alterations identified in the prenatal valproic acid model of autism spectrum disorder. *Developmental Neuroscience*, *36*(5), 371–380. https://doi.org/10.1159/000362645.

Akbarian, S., Huntsman, M. M., Kim, J. J., Tafazzoli, A., Potkin, S. G., Bunney, W. E., & Jones, E. G. (1995). $GABA_A$ receptor subunit gene expression in human prefrontal cortex: comparison of schizophrenics and controls. *Cerebral Cortex*, *5*(6), 550–560. https://doi.org/10.1093/cercor/5.6.550.

Alam, S., Westmark, C. J., & McCullagh, E. A. (2023). Diet in treatment of autism spectrum disorders. *Frontiers in Neuroscience*, *16*, 1031016. https://doi.org/10.3389/fnins.2022.1031016.

Al-Mudallal, A. S., LaManna, J. C., Lust, W. D., & Harik, S. I. (1996). Diet-induced ketosis does not cause cerebral acidosis. *Epilepsia*, *37*(3), 258–261. https://doi.org/10.1111/j.1528-1157.1996.tb00022.x.

Appleton, D. B., & DeVivo, D. C. (1974). An animal model for the ketogenic diet. *Epilepsia*, *15*(2), 211–227. https://doi.org/10.1111/j.1528-1157.1974.tb04943.x.

Ari, C., Kovács, Z., Juhasz, G., Murdun, C., Goldhagen, C. R., Koutnik, A. M., Poff, A. M., Kesl, S. L., & D'Agostino, D. P. (2016). Exogenous ketone supplements reduce anxiety-related behavior in Sprague-Dawley and Wistar albino Glaxo/Rijswijk rats. *Frontiers in Molecular Neuroscience*, *9*, 137. https://doi.org/10.3389/fnmol.2016.00137.

Atagün, M. İ., Şıkoğlu, E. M., Soykan, Ç., Serdar Süleyman, C., Ulusoy-Kaymak, S., Çayköylü, A., Algın, O., Phillips, M. L., Öngür, D., & Moore, C. M. (2017). Perisylvian GABA levels in schizophrenia and bipolar disorder. *Neuroscience Letters*, *637*(10), 70–74. https://doi.org/10.1016/j.neulet.2016.11.051.

Barbalho, C. A., Nunes-de-Souza, R. L., & Canto-de-Souza, A. (2009). Similar anxiolytic-like effects following intra-amygdala infusions of benzodiazepine receptor agonist and antagonist: Evidence for the release of an endogenous benzodiazepine inverse agonist in mice exposed to elevated plus-maze test. *Brain Research*, *1267*, 65–76. https://doi.org/10.1016/j.brainres.2009.02.042.

Benes, F. M., McSparren, J., Bird, E. D., SanGiovanni, J. P., & Vincent, S. L. (1991). Deficits in small interneurons in prefrontal and cingulate cortices of schizophrenic and schizoaffective patients. *Archives of General Psychiatry*, *48*(11), 996. https://doi.org/10.1001/archpsyc.1991.01810350036005.

Benes, F. M., Vincent, S. L., Alsterberg, G., Bird, E. D., & SanGiovanni, J. (1992). Increased GABA$_A$ receptor binding in superficial layers of cingulate cortex in schizophrenics. *The Journal of Neuroscience*, *12*(3), 924–929. https://doi.org/10.1523/JNEUROSCI.12-03-00924.1992.

Benes, F. M., Vincent, S. L., Marie, A., & Khan, Y. (1996a). Up-regulation of GABA$_A$ receptor binding on neurons of the prefrontal cortex in schizophrenic subjects. *Neuroscience*, *75*(4), 1021–1031. https://doi.org/10.1016/0306-4522(96)00328-4.

Benes, F. M., Khan, Y., Vincent, S. L., & Wickramasinghe, R. (1996b). Differences in the subregional and cellular distribution of GABA$_A$ receptor binding in the hippocampal formation of schizophrenic brain. *Synapse*, *22*(4), 338–349. https://doi.org/10.1002/(SICI)1098-2396(199604)22:4<338::AID-SYN5>3.0.CO;2-C.

Beneyto, M., Abbott, A., Hashimoto, T., & Lewis, D. A. (2011). Lamina-specific alterations in cortical GABA$_A$ receptor subunit expression in schizophrenia. *Cerebral Cortex*, *21*(5), 999–1011. https://doi.org/10.1093/cercor/bhq169.

Brady, Jr, R. O., McCarthy, J. M., Prescot, A. P., Jensen, J. E., Cooper, A. J., Cohen, B. M., Renshaw, P. F., & Öngür, D. (2013). Brain gamma-aminobutyric acid (GABA) abnormalities in bipolar disorder. *Bipolar Disorders*, *15*(4), 434–439. https://doi.org/10.1111/bdi.12074.

Brambilla, P., Perez, J., Barale, F., Schettini, G., & Soares, J. C. (2003). GABAergic dysfunction in mood disorders. *Molecular Psychiatry*, *8*(8), 721–737. https://doi.org/10.1038/sj.mp.4001362.

Brandt, A. S., Unschuld, P. G., Pradhan, S., Lim, I. A. L., Churchill, G., Harris, A. D., Hua, J., Barker, P. B., Ross, C. A., van Zijl, P. C. M., Edden, R. A. E., & Margolis, R. L. (2016). Age-related changes in anterior cingulate cortex glutamate in schizophrenia: A 1H MRS Study at 7Tesla. *Schizophrenia Research*, *172*(1–3), 101–105. https://doi.org/10.1016/j.schres.2016.02.017.

Calderón, N., Betancourt, L., Hernández, L., & Rada, P. (2017). A ketogenic diet modifies glutamate, gamma-aminobutyric acid and agmatine levels in the hippocampus of rats: A microdialysis study. *Neuroscience Letters*, *642*, 158–162. https://doi.org/10.1016/j.neulet.2017.02.014.

Campbell, I. H., & Campbell, H. (2019). Ketosis and bipolar disorder: controlled analytic study of online reports. *BJPsych Open*, *5*(4), e58. https://doi.org/10.1192/bjo.2019.49.

Campbell, I., & Campbell, H. (2020). Mechanisms of insulin resistance, mitochondrial dysfunction and the action of the ketogenic diet in bipolar disorder. Focus on the PI3K/AKT/HIF1-a pathway. *Medical Hypotheses*, *145*, 110299. https://doi.org/10.1016/j.mehy.2020.110299.

Castro, K., Baronio, D., Perry, I. S., Dos Santos, R. R., & Gottfried, C. (2017). The effect of ketogenic diet in an animal model of autism induced by prenatal exposure to

valproic acid. *Nutritional Neuroscience, 20*(6), 343–350. https://doi.org/10.1080/1028415X.2015.1133029.
Cellot, G., & Cherubini, E. (2014). GABAergic signaling as therapeutic target for autism spectrum disorders. *Frontiers in Pediatrics, 2,* 70. https://doi.org/10.3389/fped.2014.00070.
Chao, H. T., Chen, H., Samaco, R. C., Xue, M., Chahrour, M., Yoo, J., Neul, J. L., Gong, S., Lu, H. C., Heintz, N., Ekker, M., Rubenstein, J. L. R., Noebels, J. L., Rosenmund, C., & Zoghbi, H. Y. (2010). Dysfunction in GABA signalling mediates autism-like stereotypies and Rett syndrome phenotypes. *Nature, 468*(7321), 263–269. https://doi.org/10.1038/nature09582.
Chen, T., Wang, Y., Zhang, J., Wang, Z., Xu, J., Li, Y., Yang, Z., & Liu, D. (2017). Abnormal concentration of GABA and glutamate in the prefrontal cortex in schizophrenia.-An in vivo 1H-MRS study. *Shanghai Archives of Psychiatry, 29*(5), 277–286. https://doi.org/10.11919/j.issn.1002-0829.217004.
Cheng, C. M., Hicks, K., Wang, J., Eagles, D. A., & Bondy, C. A. (2004). Caloric restriction augments brain glutamic acid decarboxylase-65 and -67 expression. *Journal of Neuroscience Research, 77*(2), 270–276. https://doi.org/10.1002/jnr.20144.
Cherubini, E. 2012. Phasic GABA$_A$-Mediated Inhibition. In: *Jasper's Basic Mechanisms of the Epilepsies,* edited by Noebels, J. L., Avoli, M. & Rogawski, M. A., 1–17. Bethesda: National Center for Biotechnology Information.
Choudary, P. V., Molnar, M., Evans, S. J., Tomita, H., Li, J. Z., Vawter, M. P., Myers, R. M., Bunney, W. E., Akil, H., Watson, S. J., & Jones, E. G. (2005). Altered cortical glutamatergic and GABAergic signal transmission with glial involvement in depression. *Proceedings of the National Academy of Sciences, 102*(43), 15653–15658. https://doi.org/10.1073/pnas.0507901102.
Crestani, F., Lorez, M., Baer, K., Essrich, C., Benke, D., Laurent, J. P., Belzung, C., Fritschy, J. M., Lüscher, B., & Mohler, H. (1999). Decreased GABA$_A$-receptor clustering results in enhanced anxiety and a bias for threat cues. *Nature Neuroscience, 2*(9), 833–839. https://doi.org/10.1038/12207.
Curley, A. A., Arion, D., Volk, D. W., Asafu-Adjei, J. K., Sampson, A. R., Fish, K. N., & Lewis, D. A. (2011). Cortical deficits of glutamic acid decarboxylase 67 expression in schizophrenia: Clinical, protein, and cell type-specific features. *American Journal of Psychiatry, 168*(9), 921–929. https://doi.org/10.1176/appi.ajp.2011.11010052.
Dahlin, M., Elfving, Å., Ungerstedt, U., & Åmark, P. (2005). The ketogenic diet influences the levels of excitatory and inhibitory amino acids in the CSF in children with refractory epilepsy. *Epilepsy Research, 64*(3), 115–125. https://doi.org/10.1016/j.eplepsyres.2005.03.008.
Dai, Y., Zhao, Y., Tomi, M., Shin, B. C., Thamotharan, S., Mazarati, A., Sankar, R., Wang, E. A., Cepeda, C., Levine, M. S., Zhang, J., Frew, A., Alger, J. R., Clark, P. M., Sondhi, M., Kositamongkol, S., Leibovitch, L., & Devaskar, S. U. (2017). Sex-specific life course changes in the neuro-metabolic phenotype of Glut3 null heterozygous mice: Ketogenic diet ameliorates electroencephalographic seizures and improves sociability. *Endocrinology, 158*(4), 936–949. https://doi.org/10.1210/en.2016-1816.

Dean, B., Hussain, T., Hayes, W., Scarr, E., Kitsoulis, S., Hill, C., Opeskin, K., & Copolov, D. L. (1999). Changes in serotonin$_{2A}$ and GABA$_A$ receptors in schizophrenia. *Journal of Neurochemistry*, *72*(4), 1593–1599. https://doi.org/10.1046/j.1471-4159.1999.721593.x.

Di, J., Li, J., O'Hara, B., Alberts, I., Xiong, L., Li, J., & Li, X. (2020). The role of GABAergic neural circuits in the pathogenesis of autism spectrum disorder. *International Journal of Developmental Neuroscience*, *80*(2), 73–85. https://doi.org/10.1002/jdn.10005.

Dietch, D. M., Kerr-Gaffney, J., Hockey, M., Marx, W., Ruusunen, A., Young, A. H., Berk, M., & Mondelli, V. (2023). Efficacy of low carbohydrate and ketogenic diets in treating mood and anxiety disorders: systematic review and implications for clinical practice. *BJPsych Open*, *9*(3), e70. https://doi.org/10.1192/bjo.2023.36.

Duncan, C. E., Webster, M. J., Rothmond, D. A., Bahn, S., Elashoff, M., & Shannon Weickert, C. (2010). Prefrontal GABA$_A$ receptor α-subunit expression in normal postnatal human development and schizophrenia. *Journal of Psychiatric Research*, *44*(10), 673–681. https://doi.org/10.1016/j.jpsychires.2009.12.007.

El-Rashidy, O., El-Baz, F., El-Gendy, Y., Khalaf, R., Reda, D., & Saad, K. (2017). Ketogenic diet versus gluten free casein free diet in autistic children: a case-control study. *Metabolic Brain Disease*, *32*(6), 1935–1941. https://doi.org/10.1007/s11011-017-0088-z.

Emrich, H. M., Zerssen, D. V., Kissling, W., Möller, H. J., & Windorfer, A. (1980). Effect of sodium valproate on mania. *Archiv Für Psychiatrie Und Nervenkrankheiten*, *229*(1), 1–16. https://doi.org/10.1007/BF00343800.

Erecińska, M., Nelson, D., Daikhin, Y., & Yudkoff, M. (1996). Regulation of GABA level in rat brain synaptosomes: Fluxes through enzymes of the GABA shunt and effects of glutamate, calcium, and ketone bodies. *Journal of Neurochemistry*, *67*(6), 2325–2334. https://doi.org/10.1046/j.1471-4159.1996.67062325.x.

Evangeliou, A., Vlachonikolis, I., Mihailidou, H., Spilioti, M., Skarpalezou, A., Makaronas, N., Prokopiou, A., Christodoulou, P., Liapi-Adamidou, G., Helidonis, E., Sbyrakis, S., & Smeitink, J. (2003). Application of a ketogenic diet in children with autistic behavior: Pilot study. *Journal of Child Neurology*, *18*(2), 113–118. https://doi.org/10.1177/08830738030180020501.

Fatemi, S. H., Reutiman, T. J., Folsom, T. D., & Thuras, P. D. (2009a). GABA$_A$ receptor downregulation in brains of subjects with autism. *Journal of Autism and Developmental Disorders*, *39*(2), 223–230. https://doi.org/10.1007/s10803-008-0646-7.

Fatemi, S. H., Folsom, T. D., Reutiman, T. J., & Thuras, P. D. (2009b). Expression of GABA$_B$ receptors is altered in brains of subjects with autism. *The Cerebellum*, *8*(1), 64–69. https://doi.org/10.1007/s12311-008-0075-3.

Fatemi, S. H., Folsom, T. D., & Thuras, P. D. (2011). Deficits in GABA$_B$ receptor system in schizophrenia and mood disorders: A postmortem study. *Schizophrenia Research*, *128*(1–3), 37–43. https://doi.org/10.1016/j.schres.2010.12.025.

Fatemi, S. H., Folsom, T. D., & Thuras, P. D. (2017). GABA$_A$ and GABA$_B$ receptor dysregulation in superior frontal cortex of subjects with schizophrenia and bipolar disorder. *Synapse*, *71*(7). https://doi.org/10.1002/syn.21973.

Fedorovich, S., Voronina, P., & Waseem, T. (2018). Ketogenic diet versus ketoacidosis: what determines the influence of ketone bodies on neurons? *Neural Regeneration Research*, *13*(12), 2060. https://doi.org/10.4103/1673-5374.241442.

Gilbert-Jaramillo, J., Vargas-Pico, D., Espinosa-Mendoza, T., Falk, S., Llanos-Fernandez, K., Guerrero-Haro, J., Orellana-Roman, C., Poveda-Loor, C., Valdevila-Figueira, J., & Palmer, C. (2018). The effects of the ketogenic diet on psychiatric symptomatology, weight and metabolic dysfunction in schizophrenia patients. *Clinical Nutrition and Metabolism*, *1*(1), 1–5. https://doi.org/10.15761/CNM.1000105.

Glausier, J. R., Kimoto, S., Fish, K. N., & Lewis, D. A. (2015). Lower glutamic acid decarboxylase 65-kDa isoform messenger RNA and protein levels in the prefrontal cortex in schizoaffective disorder but not schizophrenia. *Biological Psychiatry*, *77*(2), 167–176. https://doi.org/10.1016/j.biopsych.2014.05.010.

Gold, B. I., Bowers, M. B., Roth, R. H., & Sweeney, D. W. (1980). GABA levels in CSF of patients with psychiatric disorders. *American Journal of Psychiatry*, *137*(3), 362–364. https://doi.org/10.1176/ajp.137.3.362.

Goto, N., Yoshimura, R., Kakeda, S., Moriya, J., Hori, H., Hayashi, K., Ikenouchi-Sugita, A., Nakano-Umene, W., Katsuki, A., Nishimura, J., Korogi, Y., & Nakamura, J. (2010). No alterations of brain GABA after 6 months of treatment with atypical antipsychotic drugs in early-stage first-episode schizophrenia. *Progress in Neuro-Psychopharmacology and Biological Psychiatry*, *34*(8), 1480–1483. https://doi.org/10.1016/j.pnpbp.2010.08.007.

Granados-Rojas, L., Jerónimo-Cruz, K., Juárez-Zepeda, T. E., Tapia-Rodríguez, M., Tovar, A. R., Rodríguez-Jurado, R., Carmona-Aparicio, L., Cárdenas-Rodríguez, N., Coballase-Urrutia, E., Ruíz-García, M., & Durán, P. (2020). Ketogenic diet provided during three months increases KCC2 expression but Not NKCC1 in the rat dentate gyrus. *Frontiers in Neuroscience*, *14*, 673. https://doi.org/10.3389/fnins.2020.00673.

Guidotti, A., Auta, J., Davis, J. M., Gerevini, V. D., Dwivedi, Y., Grayson, D. R., Impagnatiello, F., Pandey, G., Pesold, C., Sharma, R., Uzunov, D., & Costa, E. (2000). Decrease in reelin and glutamic acid decarboxylase67 (GAD67) expression in schizophrenia and bipolar disorder. *Archives of General Psychiatry*, *57*(11), 1061–1069. https://doi.org/10.1001/archpsyc.57.11.1061.

Gzieło, K., Janeczko, K., Węglarz, W., Jasiński, K., Kłodowski, K., & Setkowicz, Z. (2020). MRI spectroscopic and tractography studies indicate consequences of long-term ketogenic diet. *Brain Structure and Function*, *225*(7), 2077–2089. https://doi.org/10.1007/s00429-020-02111-9.

Hashimoto, T., Bazmi, H. H., Mirnics, K., Wu, Q., Sampson, A. R., & Lewis, D. A. (2008a). Conserved regional patterns of GABA-related transcript expression in the neocortex of subjects with schizophrenia. *American Journal of Psychiatry*, *165*(4), 479–489. https://doi.org/10.1176/appi.ajp.2007.07081223.

Hashimoto, T., Arion, D., Unger, T., Maldonado-Avilés, J. G., Morris, H. M., Volk, D. W., Mirnics, K., & Lewis, D. A. (2008b). Alterations in GABA-related transcriptome in the dorsolateral prefrontal cortex of subjects with schizophrenia. *Molecular Psychiatry*, *13*(2), 147–161. https://doi.org/10.1038/sj.mp.4002011.

Hasler, G. (2010). Pathophysiology of depression: do we have any solid evidence of interest to clinicians? *World Psychiatry*, *9*(3), 155–161. https://doi.org/10.1002/j.2051-5545.2010.tb00298.x.

Hellsten, K. S., Sinkkonen, S. T., Hyde, T. M., Kleinman, J. E., Särkioja, T., Maksimow, A., Uusi-Oukari, M., & Korpi, E. R. (2010). Human locus coeruleus neurons express the GABA$_A$ receptor γ2 subunit gene and produce benzodiazepine binding. *Neuroscience Letters*, *477*(2), 77–81. https://doi.org/10.1016/j.neulet.2010.04.035.

Hodges, H., Fealko, C., & Soares, N. (2020). Autism spectrum disorder: definition, epidemiology, causes, and clinical evaluation. *Translational Pediatrics*, *9*(S1), S55–S65. https://doi.org/10.21037/tp.2019.09.09.

Höhn, S., Dozières-Puyravel, B., & Auvin, S. (2019). History of dietary treatment from Wilder's hypothesis to the first open studies in the 1920s. *Epilepsy & Behavior*, *101*, 106588. https://doi.org/10.1016/j.yebeh.2019.106588.

Huntsman, M. M., Tran, B. V., Potkin, S. G., Bunney, W. E., & Jones, E. G. (1998). Altered ratios of alternatively spliced long and short γ2 subunit mRNAs of the γ-amino butyrate type A receptor in prefrontal cortex of schizophrenics. *Proceedings of the National Academy of Sciences*, *95*(25), 15066–15071. https://doi.org/10.1073/pnas.95.25.15066.

Impagnatiello, F., Guidotti, A. R., Pesold, C., Dwivedi, Y., Caruncho, H., Pisu, M. G., Uzunov, D. P., Smalheiser, N. R., Davis, J. M., Pandey, G. N., Pappas, G. D., Tueting, P., Sharma, R. P., & Costa, E. (1998). A decrease of reelin expression as a putative vulnerability factor in schizophrenia. *Proceedings of the National Academy of Sciences*, *95*(26), 15718–15723. https://doi.org/10.1073/pnas.95.26.15718.

Ishikawa, M., Mizukami, K., Iwakiri, M., Hidaka, S., & Asada, T. (2004). Immunohistochemical and immunoblot study of GABA$_A$ α1 and β2/3 subunits in the prefrontal cortex of subjects with schizophrenia and bipolar disorder. *Neuroscience Research*, *50*(1), 77–84. https://doi.org/10.1016/j.neures.2004.06.006.

Ishikawa, M., Mizukami, K., Iwakiri, M., & Asada, T. (2005). Immunohistochemical and immunoblot analysis of γ-aminobutyric acid B receptor in the prefrontal cortex of subjects with schizophrenia and bipolar disorder. *Neuroscience Letters*, *383*(3), 272–277. https://doi.org/10.1016/j.neulet.2005.04.025.

Joshi, D., Fung, S. J., Rothwell, A., & Weickert, C. S. (2012). Higher gamma-aminobutyric acid neuron density in the white matter of orbital frontal cortex in schizophrenia. *Biological Psychiatry*, *72*(9), 725–733. https://doi.org/10.1016/j.biopsych.2012.06.021.

Kahn, R. S., Sommer, I. E., Murray, R. M., Meyer-Lindenberg, A., Weinberger, D. R., Cannon, T. D., O'Donovan, M., Correll, C. U., Kane, J. M., van Os, J., & Insel, T. R. (2015). Schizophrenia. *Nature Reviews Disease Primers*, *1*(1), 15067. https://doi.org/10.1038/nrdp.2015.67.

Kalueff, A. V., & Nutt, D. J. (2007). Role of GABA in anxiety and depression. *Depression and Anxiety*, *24*(7), 495–517. https://doi.org/10.1002/da.20262.

Kaufman, R. E., Ostacher, M. J., Marks, E. H., Simon, N. M., Sachs, G. S., Jensen, J. E., Renshaw, P. F., & Pollack, M. H. (2009). Brain GABA levels in patients with bipolar disorder. *Progress in Neuro-Psychopharmacology and Biological Psychiatry*, *33*(3), 427–434. https://doi.org/10.1016/j.pnpbp.2008.12.025.

Kegeles, L. S., Mao, X., Stanford, A. D., Girgis, R., Ojeil, N., Xu, X., Gil, R., Slifstein, M., Abi-Dargham, A., Lisanby, S. H., & Shungu, D. C. (2012). Elevated prefrontal cortex γ-aminobutyric acid and glutamate-glutamine levels in schizophrenia measured in vivo with proton magnetic resonance spectroscopy. *Archives of General Psychiatry*, *69*(5), 449–459. https://doi.org/10.1001/archgenpsychiatry.2011.1519.

Kerub, O., Haas, E., Menashe, I., Davidovitch, N., & Meiri, G. (2018). Autism spectrum disorder: evolution of disorder definition, risk factors and demographic characteristics in Israel. *The Israel Medical Association Journal*, *20*, 576–581.

Klumpers, U. M. H., Veltman, D. J., Drent, M. L., Boellaard, R., Comans, E. F. I., Meynen, G., Lammertsma, A. A., & Hoogendijk, W. J. G. (2010). Reduced parahippocampal and lateral temporal $GABA_A$-[^{11}C]flumazenil binding in major depression: preliminary results. *European Journal of Nuclear Medicine and Molecular Imaging*, *37*(3), 565–574. https://doi.org/10.1007/s00259-009-1292-9.

Kobayashi, M., Hayashi, Y., Fujimoto, Y., & Matsuoka, I. (2018). Decreased parvalbumin and somatostatin neurons in medial prefrontal cortex in BRINP1-KO mice. *Neuroscience Letters*, *683*, 82–88. https://doi.org/10.1016/j.neulet.2018.06.050.

Konradi, C., Yang, C. K., Zimmerman, E. I., Lohmann, K. M., Gresch, P., Pantazopoulos, H., Berretta, S., & Heckers, S. (2011). Hippocampal interneurons are abnormal in schizophrenia. *Schizophrenia Research*, *131*(1–3), 165–173. https://doi.org/10.1016/j.schres.2011.06.007.

Kraeuter, A. K., Loxton, H., Lima, B. C., Rudd, D., & Sarnyai, Z. (2015). Ketogenic diet reverses behavioral abnormalities in an acute NMDA receptor hypofunction model of schizophrenia. *Schizophrenia Research*, *169*(1–3), 491–493. https://doi.org/10.1016/j.schres.2015.10.041.

Kraeuter, A. K., van den Buuse, M., & Sarnyai, Z. (2019). Ketogenic diet prevents impaired prepulse inhibition of startle in an acute NMDA receptor hypofunction model of schizophrenia. *Schizophrenia Research*, *206*, 244–250. https://doi.org/10.1016/j.schres.2018.11.011.

Kraft, B. D., & Westman, E. C. (2009). Schizophrenia, gluten, and low-carbohydrate, ketogenic diets: a case report and review of the literature. *Nutrition & Metabolism*, *6*(1), 10. https://doi.org/10.1186/1743-7075-6-10.

Lauritzen, K. H., Hasan-Olive, M. M., Regnell, C. E., Kleppa, L., Scheibye-Knudsen, M., Gjedde, A., Klungland, A., Bohr, V. A., Storm-Mathisen, J., & Bergersen, L. H. (2016). A ketogenic diet accelerates neurodegeneration in mice with induced mitochondrial DNA toxicity in the forebrain. *Neurobiology of Aging*, *48*, 34–47. https://doi.org/10.1016/j.neurobiolaging.2016.08.005.

Lawrence, Y. A., Kemper, T. L., Bauman, M. L., & Blatt, G. J. (2010). Parvalbumin-, calbindin-, and calretinin-immunoreactive hippocampal interneuron density in autism. *Acta Neurologica Scandinavica*, *121*(2), 99–108. https://doi.org/10.1111/j.1600-0404.2009.01234.x.

Lee, R. W. Y., Corley, M. J., Pang, A., Arakaki, G., Abbott, L., Nishimoto, M., Miyamoto, R., Lee, E., Yamamoto, S., Maunakea, A. K., Lum-Jones, A., & Wong, M. (2018). A modified ketogenic gluten-free diet with MCT improves behavior in children with autism spectrum disorder. *Physiology & Behavior*, *188*, 205–211. https://doi.org/10.1016/j.physbeh.2018.02.006.

Lord, C., Elsabbagh, M., Baird, G., & Veenstra-Vanderweele, J. (2018). Autism spectrum disorder. *Lancet*, *392*(10146), 508–520. https://doi.org/10.1016/S0140-6736(18)31129-2.

Luscher, B., & Fuchs, T. (2015). GABAergic control of depression-related brain states. *Advances in Pharmacology*, *73*, 97–144. https://doi.org/10.1016/bs.apha.2014.11.003.

Maldonado-Avilés, J. G., Curley, A. A., Hashimoto, T., Morrow, A. L., Ramsey, A. J., O'Donnell, P., Volk, D. W., & Lewis, D. A. (2009). Altered markers of tonic inhibition in the dorsolateral prefrontal cortex of subjects with schizophrenia. *American Journal of Psychiatry*, *166*(4), 450–459. https://doi.org/10.1176/appi.ajp.2008.08101484.

Maroney, M. (2020). An update on current treatment strategies and emerging agents for the management of schizophrenia. *The American Journal of Managed Care*, *26*(3 Suppl), S55–S61. https://doi.org/10.37765/ajmc.2020.43012.

Marsman, A., Mandl, R. C. W., Klomp, D. W. J., Bohlken, M. M., Boer, V. O., Andreychenko, A., Cahn, W., Kahn, R. S., Luijten, P. R., & Hulshoff Pol, H. E. (2014). GABA and glutamate in schizophrenia: A 7 T 1H-MRS study. *NeuroImage: Clinical*, *6*, 398–407. https://doi.org/10.1016/j.nicl.2014.10.005.

McDonald, T. J. W., & Cervenka, M. C. (2018). Ketogenic diets for adult neurological disorders. *Neurotherapeutics*, *15*(4), 1018–1031. https://doi.org/10.1007/s13311-018-0666-8.

McDougall, A., Bayley, M., & Munce, S. E. (2018). The ketogenic diet as a treatment for traumatic brain injury: a scoping review. *Brain Injury*, *32*(4), 416–422. https://doi.org/10.1080/02699052.2018.1429025.

Melø, T. M., Nehlig, A., & Sonnewald, U. (2006). Neuronal-glial interactions in rats fed a ketogenic diet. *Neurochemistry International*, *48*(6–7), 498–507. https://doi.org/10.1016/j.neuint.2005.12.037.

Möhler, H. (2012). The GABA system in anxiety and depression and its therapeutic potential. *Neuropharmacology*, *62*(1), 42–53. https://doi.org/10.1016/j.neuropharm.2011.08.040.

Moyer, C. E., Delevich, K. M., Fish, K. N., Asafu-Adjei, J. K., Sampson, A. R., Dorph-Petersen, K. A., Lewis, D. A., & Sweet, R. A. (2012). Reduced glutamate decarboxylase 65 protein within primary auditory cortex inhibitory boutons in schizophrenia. *Biological Psychiatry*, *72*(9), 734–743. https://doi.org/10.1016/j.biopsych.2012.04.010.

Mu, C., Corley, M. J., Lee, R. W. Y., Wong, M., Pang, A., Arakaki, G., Miyamoto, R., Rho, J. M., Mickiewicz, B., Dowlatabadi, R., Vogel, H. J., Korchemagin, Y., & Shearer, J. (2020). Metabolic framework for the improvement of autism spectrum disorders by a modified ketogenic diet: A pilot study. *Journal of Proteome Research*, *19*(1), 382–390. https://doi.org/10.1021/acs.jproteome.9b00581.

Murphy, P., Likhodii, S., Nylen, K., & Burnham, W. M. (2004). The antidepressant properties of the ketogenic diet. *Biological Psychiatry*, *56*(12), 981–983. https://doi.org/10.1016/j.biopsych.2004.09.019.

Napoli, E., Dueñas, N., & Giulivi, C. (2014). Potential therapeutic use of the ketogenic diet in autism spectrum disorders. *Frontiers in Pediatrics*, *2*, 69. https://doi.org/10.3389/fped.2014.00069.

National Institutes of Health. (2021a, October). *Anxiety disorders*. Https://www.Nimh.Nih.Gov/Health/Topics/Anxiety-Disorders.

National Institutes of Health. (2021b, October). *Bipolar disorder*. Https://www.Nimh.Nih.Gov/Health/Topics/Bipolar-Disorder.

Nuss, P. (2015). Anxiety disorders and GABA neurotransmission: a disturbance of modulation. *Neuropsychiatric Disease and Treatment*, *11*, 165-175. https://doi.org/10.2147/NDT.S58841.

Oblak, A., Gibbs, T. T., & Blatt, G. J. (2009). Decreased $GABA_A$ receptors and benzodiazepine binding sites in the anterior cingulate cortex in autism. *Autism Research*, *2*(4), 205–219. https://doi.org/10.1002/aur.88.

Oblak, A. L., Gibbs, T. T., & Blatt, G. J. (2010). Decreased $GABA_B$ receptors in the cingulate cortex and fusiform gyrus in autism. *Journal of Neurochemistry*, *114*(5), 1414–1423. https://doi.org/10.1111/j.1471-4159.2010.06858.x.

Ohnuma, T., Augood, S. J., Arai, H., McKenna, P. J., & Emson, P. C. (1999). Measurement of GABAergic parameters in the prefrontal cortex in schizophrenia: focus on GABA content, $GABA_A$ receptor α-1 subunit messenger RNA and human GABA transporter-1 (hGAT-1) messenger RNA expression. *Neuroscience*, *93*(2), 441–448. https://doi.org/10.1016/S0306-4522(99)00189-X.

Olmos-Serrano, J. L., Paluszkiewicz, S. M., Martin, B. S., Kaufmann, W. E., Corbin, J. G., & Huntsman, M. M. (2010). Defective GABAergic neurotransmission and pharmacological rescue of neuronal hyperexcitability in the amygdala in a mouse model of fragile X syndrome. *Journal of Neuroscience*, *30*(29), 9929–9938. https://doi.org/10.1523/JNEUROSCI.1714-10.2010.

Pacheco, A., Easterling, W. S., & Pryer, M. W. (1965). A pilot study of the ketogenic diet in schizophrenia. *American Journal of Psychiatry*, *121*(11), 1110–1111. https://doi.org/10.1176/ajp.121.11.1110.

Palmer, C. M. (2017). Ketogenic diet in the treatment of schizoaffective disorder: Two case studies. *Schizophrenia Research*, *189*, 208–209. https://doi.org/10.1016/j.schres.2017.01.053.

Palmer, C. M., Gilbert-Jaramillo, J., & Westman, E. C. (2019). The ketogenic diet and remission of psychotic symptoms in schizophrenia: Two case studies. *Schizophrenia Research*, *208*, 439–440. https://doi.org/10.1016/j.schres.2019.03.019.

Phelps, J. R., Siemers, S. V., & El-Mallakh, R. S. (2013). The ketogenic diet for type II bipolar disorder. *Neurocase*, *19*(5), 423–426. https://doi.org/10.1080/13554794.2012.690421.

Pizzarelli, R., & Cherubini, E. (2011). Alterations of GABAergic signaling in autism spectrum disorders. *Neural Plasticity*, *2011*, 297153. doi: 10.1155/2011/297153. https://doi.org/10.1155/2011/297153.

Price, R. B., Shungu, D. C., Mao, X., Nestadt, P., Kelly, C., Collins, K. A., Murrough, J. W., Charney, D. S., & Mathew, S. J. (2009). Amino acid neurotransmitters assessed by proton magnetic resonance spectroscopy: Relationship to treatment resistance in major depressive disorder. *Biological Psychiatry, 65*(9), 792–800. https://doi.org/10.1016/j.biopsych.2008.10.025.

Puts, N. A. J., Wodka, E. L., Harris, A. D., Crocetti, D., Tommerdahl, M., Mostofsky, S. H., & Edden, R. A. E. (2017). Reduced GABA and altered somatosensory function in children with autism spectrum disorder. *Autism Research, 10*(4), 608–619. https://doi.org/10.1002/aur.1691.

Ricci, A., Idzikowski, M. A., Soares, C. N., & Brietzke, E. (2020). Exploring the mechanisms of action of the antidepressant effect of the ketogenic diet. *Reviews in the Neurosciences, 31*(6), 637–648. https://doi.org/10.1515/revneuro-2019-0073.

Rogawski, M. A., Löscher, W., & Rho, J. M. (2016). Mechanisms of action of antiseizure drugs and the ketogenic diet. *Cold Spring Harbor Perspectives in Medicine, 6*(5), a022780. https://doi.org/10.1101/cshperspect.a022780.

Rojas, D. C., Singel, D., Steinmetz, S., Hepburn, S., & Brown, M. S. (2014). Decreased left perisylvian GABA concentration in children with autism and unaffected siblings. *NeuroImage, 86*, 28–34. https://doi.org/10.1016/j.neuroimage.2013.01.045.

Rowland, L. M., Kontson, K., West, J., Edden, R. A., Zhu, H., Wijtenburg, S. A., Holcomb, H. H., & Barker, P. B. (2013). In vivo measurements of glutamate, GABA, and NAAG in schizophrenia. *Schizophrenia Bulletin, 39*(5), 1096–1104. https://doi.org/10.1093/schbul/sbs092.

Ruskin, D. N., Svedova, J., Cote, J. L., Sandau, U., Rho, J. M., Kawamura, M., Boison, D., & Masino, S. A. (2013). Ketogenic diet improves core symptoms of autism in BTBR mice. *Plos One, 8*(6), e65021. https://doi.org/10.1371/journal.pone.0065021.

Ruskin, D. N., Murphy, M. I., Slade, S. L., & Masino, S. A. (2017). Ketogenic diet improves behaviors in a maternal immune activation model of autism spectrum disorder. *Plos One, 12*(2), e0171643. https://doi.org/10.1371/journal.pone.0171643.

Sarnyai, Z., Kraeuter, A. K., & Palmer, C. M. (2019). Ketogenic diet for schizophrenia. *Current Opinion in Psychiatry, 32*(5), 394–401. https://doi.org/10.1097/YCO.0000000000000535.

Seeman, P., & Kapur, S. (2000). Schizophrenia: More dopamine, more D$_2$ receptors. *Proceedings of the National Academy of Sciences, 97*(14), 7673–7675. https://doi.org/10.1073/pnas.97.14.7673.

Shaafi, S., Mahmoudi, J., Pashapour, A., Farhoudi, M., Sadigh-Eteghad, S., & Akbari, H. (2014). Ketogenic diet provides neuroprotective effects against ischemic stroke neuronal damages. *Advanced Pharmaceutical Bulletin, 4*(Suppl 2), 479–481. https://doi.org/10.5681/apb.2014.071.

Shen, Q., Lal, R., Luellen, B. A., Earnheart, J. C., Andrews, A. M., & Luscher, B. (2010). γ-Aminobutyric acid-type A receptor deficits cause hypothalamic-pituitary-adrenal axis hyperactivity and antidepressant drug sensitivity reminiscent of melancholic forms of depression. *Biological Psychiatry, 68*(6), 512–520. https://doi.org/10.1016/j.biopsych.2010.04.024.

Sigvard, A. K., Bojesen, K. B., Ambrosen, K. S., Nielsen, M. Ø., Gjedde, A., Tangmose, K., Kumakura, Y., Edden, R., Fuglø, D., Jensen, L. T., Rostrup, E., Ebdrup, B. H., & Glenthøj, B. Y. (2023). Dopamine synthesis capacity and GABA and glutamate levels separate antipsychotic-naïve patients with first-episode psychosis from healthy control subjects in a multimodal prediction model. *Biological Psychiatry Global Open Science, 3*(3), 500–509. https://doi.org/10.1016/j.bpsgos.2022.05.004.

Sinkkonen, S. T., Homanics, G. E., & Korpi, E. R. (2003). Mouse models of Angelman syndrome, a neurodevelopmental disorder, display different brain regional GABA$_A$ receptor alterations. *Neuroscience Letters, 340*(3), 205–208. https://doi.org/10.1016/S0304-3940(03)00123-X.

Stafstrom, C. E., & Rho, J. M. (2012). The ketogenic diet as a treatment paradigm for diverse neurological disorders. *Frontiers in Pharmacology, 3*, 59. https://doi.org/10.3389/fphar.2012.00059.

Sussman, D., Germann, J., & Henkelman, M. (2015). Gestational ketogenic diet programs brain structure and susceptibility to depression & anxiety in the adult mouse offspring. *Brain and Behavior, 5*(2), e00300. https://doi.org/10.1002/brb3.300.

Suzuki, Y., Takahashi, H., Fukuda, M., Hino, H., Kobayashi, K., Tanaka, J., & Ishii, E. (2009). β-hydroxybutyrate alters GABA-transaminase activity in cultured astrocytes. *Brain Research, 1268*, 17–23. https://doi.org/10.1016/j.brainres.2009.02.074.

Thompson, M., Weickert, C. S., Wyatt, E., & Webster, M. J. (2009). Decreased glutamic acid decarboxylase67 mRNA expression in multiple brain areas of patients with schizophrenia and mood disorders. *Journal of Psychiatric Research, 43*(11), 970–977. https://doi.org/10.1016/j.jpsychires.2009.02.005.

Tregellas, J. R., Smucny, J., Legget, K. T., & Stevens, K. E. (2015). Effects of a ketogenic diet on auditory gating in DBA/2 mice: A proof-of-concept study. *Schizophrenia Research, 169*(1–3), 351–354. https://doi.org/10.1016/j.schres.2015.09.022.

Vargas, C., Tannhauser, M., & Barros, H. M. T. (1998). Dissimilar effects of lithium and valproic acid on GABA and glutamine concentrations in rat cerebrospinal fluid. *General Pharmacology: The Vascular System, 30*(4), 601–604. https://doi.org/10.1016/S0306-3623(97)00328-5.

Verpeut, J. L., DiCicco-Bloom, E., & Bello, N. T. (2016). Ketogenic diet exposure during the juvenile period increases social behaviors and forebrain neural activation in adult Engrailed 2 null mice. *Physiology & Behavior, 161*, 90–98. https://doi.org/10.1016/j.physbeh.2016.04.001.

Volk, D. W., Austin, M. C., Pierri, J. N., Sampson, A. R., & Lewis, D. A. (2001). GABA Benes, F. M., Vincent, S. L., Alsterberg, G., Bird, E., & San Giovanni, J. (1992) transporter-1 mRNA in the prefrontal cortex in schizophrenia: Decreased expression in a subset of neurons. *American Journal of Psychiatry, 158*(2), 256–265. https://doi.org/10.1176/appi.ajp.158.2.256.

Volk, D. W., Pierri, J. N., Fritschy, J. M., Auh, S., Sampson, A. R., & Lewis, D. A. (2002). Reciprocal alterations in pre- and postsynaptic inhibitory markers at chandelier cell inputs to pyramidal neurons in schizophrenia. *Cerebral Cortex, 12*(10), 1063–1070. https://doi.org/10.1093/cercor/12.10.1063.

Wang, Z. J., Bergqvist, C., Hunter, J. V, Jin, D., Wang, D. J., Wehrli, S., & Zimmerman, R. A. (2003). In vivo measurement of brain metabolites using two-dimensional double-quantum MR spectroscopy-exploration of GABA levels in a ketogenic diet. *Magnetic Resonance in Medicine, 49*(4), 615–619. https://doi.org/10.1002/mrm.10429.

Wang, A. Y., Lohmann, K. M., Yang, C. K., Zimmerman, E. I., Pantazopoulos, H., Herring, N., Berretta, S., Heckers, S., & Konradi, C. (2011). Bipolar disorder type 1 and schizophrenia are accompanied by decreased density of parvalbumin- and somatostatin-positive interneurons in the parahippocampal region. *Acta Neuropathologica*, *122*(5), 615–626. https://doi.org/10.1007/s00401-011-0881-4.

Wheless, J. W. (2008). History of the ketogenic diet. *Epilepsia*, *49*(s8), 3–5. https://doi.org/10.1111/j.1528-1167.2008.01821.x.

Włodarczyk, A., Cubała, W. J., & Wielewicka, A. (2020). Ketogenic diet: A dietary modification as an anxiolytic approach? *Nutrients*, *12*(12), 3822. https://doi.org/10.3390/nu12123822.

Włodarczyk, A., Cubała, W. J., & Stawicki, M. (2021). Ketogenic diet for depression: A potential dietary regimen to maintain euthymia? *Progress in Neuro-Psychopharmacology and Biological Psychiatry*, *109*, 110257. https://doi.org/10.1016/j.pnpbp.2021.110257.

Won, E., & Kim, Y. K. (2017). An oldie but goodie: Lithium in the teatment of bipolar disorder through neuroprotective and neurotrophic mechanisms. *International Journal of Molecular Sciences*, *18*(12), 2679. https://doi.org/10.3390/ijms18122679.

World Health Organization. Depression. Accessed October 18, 2021. https://www.who.int/health-topics/depression#tab=tab_3.

Yip, J., Soghomonian, J. J., & Blatt, G. J. (2007). Decreased GAD67 mRNA levels in cerebellar Purkinje cells in autism: pathophysiological implications. *Acta Neuropathologica*, *113*(5), 559–568. https://doi.org/10.1007/s00401-006-0176-3.

Yu, B., Ozveren, R., & Sheti, S. (2017). The use of a low carbohydrate, ketogenic diet in bipolar disorder: systematic review. *Research Square*. https://doi.org/10.21203/rs.3.rs-334453/v1.

Yudkoff, M., Daikhin, Y., Nissim, I., Lazarow, A., & Nissim, I. (2001). Brain amino acid metabolism and ketosis. *Journal of Neuroscience Research*, *66*(2), 272–281. https://doi.org/10.1002/jnr.1221.

Yudkoff, M., Daikhin, Y., Nissim, I., Horyn, O., Lazarow, A., Luhovyy, B., Wehrli, S., & Nissim, I. (2005). Response of brain amino acid metabolism to ketosis. *Neurochemistry International*, *47*(1–2), 119–128. https://doi.org/10.1016/j.neuint.2005.04.014.

Zarnowska, I., Chrapko, B., Gwizda, G., Nocun, A., Mitosek-Szewczyk, K., & Gasior, M. (2018). Therapeutic use of carbohydrate-restricted diets in an autistic child; a case report of clinical and 18FDG PET findings. *Metabolic Brain Disease*, *33*(4), 1187–1192. https://doi.org/10.1007/s11011-018-0219-1.

Zhang, Z. J., & Reynolds, G. P. (2002). A selective decrease in the relative density of parvalbumin-immunoreactive neurons in the hippocampus in schizophrenia. *Schizophrenia Research*, *55*(1–2), 1–10. https://doi.org/10.1016/S0920-9964(01)00188-8.

Chapter 5

The Ketogenic Diet and Cancer Prevention

Fernando Gatica[1]
Noél Gallardo[1]
Eric Uribe[1]
Diana Flores[1]
Vanessa Mena[1]
Amalia Alejo[2,3]
David Vázquez[1]
and Carmen Rubio[1,*]

[1]Departamento de Neurofisiología, Instituto Nacional de Neurología y Neurocirugía Manuel Velasco Suárez, Mexico City, Mexico
[2]Laboratorio de Dolor y Analgesia, Departamento de Farmacobiología, CINVESTAV Sede Sur, Mexico City, Mexico
[3]Departamento de Neurología y Psiquiatría. Instituto Nacional de Ciencias Médicas y Nutrición Salvador Zubirán, Mexico City, Mexico

Abstract

The ketogenic diet (KD) consists of the consumption of foods rich in fat with the aim of achieving nutritional ketosis. Diet plays an important role in people's health; it can prevent the development of diseases and have positive effects in the treatment of some diseases. Originally, KD was introduced to treat drug-resistant epileptic encephalopathies; however, its benefits have now spread to other chronic degenerative diseases such as cancer, including brain cancer, such as gliomas. Since the establishment

---

[*] Corresponding Author's Email: macaru4@yahoo.com.mx.

In: The Ketogenic Diet Reexamined
Editors: Leticia Granados-Rojas and Carmen Rubio
ISBN: 979-8-89113-543-7
© 2024 Nova Science Publishers, Inc.

of hallmarks of cancer, the location of cancer targets has been facilitated, among these features are the mechanisms of the anticancer properties of KD. KD can modify the microenvironment of cancer cells through energetic alterations (related to the Warburg effect), anti-inflammatory effects via inflammasome, and epigenetic changes secondary to DNA methylation and micro-RNA (miR) control. KD has also been found to be useful by increasing the sensitivity to chemotherapy and radiation therapy in certain malignant tumors, such as glioblastomas. However, a large field of study exists to explore between KD and cancer.

Keywords: ketogenic diet, cancer prevention, inflammation, ketone bodies

Acronyms

AcAc	Acetoacetate
ASC	Caspase recruitment domain
ATP	Adenosine triphosphate
BHB	β-hydroxybutyrate
DAMPs	Damage-associated molecular patterns
GLOBOCAN	Global Cancer Observatory
HMG-CoA	Hydroxymethylglutaril-CoA
IL-1R	IL-1 receptor
KD	Ketogenic diet
miR	micro-RNA
NF-κB	Nuclear factor κB
NLR	NOD-like protein
NLRP3	NOD-like receptor pyrin domain-containing 3
OXPHOS	mitochondrial oxidative phosphorylation
PAMPs	Pathogen-associated molecular patterns
PI3K	Phosphatidylinositol 3-kinase
pRB	Retinoblastoma protein
TCA	Tricarboxylic acid cycle
TLR	Toll-like receptor
TNF	Tumor necrosis factor
TOR	Target of Rapamycin

Introduction

The KD is a non-pharmacological therapeutic intervention aimed at producing a state of ketosis. Ketosis consists of increased levels of ketone bodies in the blood such as β-hydroxybutyrate (BHB), acetoacetate (AcAc), or acetone (Zhu et al., 2022). Since 400 B. C. dietary modifications have been proposed as an adjunct to the management of chronic diseases such as epilepsy, however, it was not until a little over a century ago that it was introduced as a formal therapy in refractory epilepsy. In recent years, the benefits of KD have been demonstrated in some other pathologies such as cardiovascular disease, obesity, diabetes, and cancer (Wheless, 2008). Furthermore, it is suggested that prolonged use of KD may induce modifications in the microbiome and epigenetic changes. However, it is noted that these alterations in molecular signaling are obtained under strict KD therapeutic schemes in which fat intake represents up to 90% of macronutrients ingested (Dowis & Banga, 2021).

The term 'cancer' has been used since ancient times; it is believed that Hippocrates coined it from the Greek *karkinos*, relative to the movements of a crab that resembles this by its invasion and proliferation characteristics. However, tumors may have existed in other species before the appearance of the human race (Hajdu, 2011). The importance of cancer lies in the fact that today has the highest rates of morbidity and mortality worldwide. According to the Global Cancer Observatory (GLOBOCAN) 2020 data, every year about 20 million new cases of malignant tumors are detected and almost 10 million people die each year due to the consequences of cancer. It is estimated that in the coming years cancer will become the first cause of death worldwide, surpassing cardiovascular disease (Sung et al., 2021).

In order of frequency, breast cancer (11.7%), lung cancer (11.4%), colorectal cancer (10%), prostate cancer (7.3%), and stomach cancer (5.6%) correspond to the five types of cancer with the highest incidence worldwide. In particular, the etiopathogenesis of the lifestyle of these neoplasms plays a very important role, highlighting the fact that the Western diet is nutritionally poor, with high consumption of carbohydrates and junk food. This is reflected in the incidence of cancer in geographical areas such as Australia, North America, and Western Europe. Because of all this, dietary intervention in cancer prevention is of the utmost relevance (Sung et al., 2021).

Vitamin intake has been recommended as an anti-cancer measure for several decades due to its antioxidant properties. However, in recent years a line of research has been opened that could suggest that states of ketosis caused by fasting, caloric restriction or KD could be useful in cancer prevention. It seems that the molecular target of these mechanisms lies in the energy metabolism of cells, local and systemic inflammation, as well as genetic modifications of precancerous cells.

Pathogenesis

Defining the pathophysiology of cancer is extremely complex, even more so, considering that almost any tissue or organ can develop this pathology. A neoplasm is the result of excessive and disordered proliferation and growth of cells in a tissue. However, certain features differentiate a malignant tumor from a malignant neoplasm. The first is the degree of differentiation or anaplasia of healthy cells because, while a benign tumor is well differentiated and has slow growth, malignant tumors have anaplastic cells with rapid growth. Local invasion with infiltration into the surrounding tissue is another defining feature of cancer. Finally, metastasis, which consists of the ability to spread to organs distant from the primary tumor, is another distinguishing feature of malignancies; however, this feature is debatable in brain gliomas and basal cell carcinomas, which present the histopathological findings of malignant neoplasms without performing distant metastasis (Hanahan & Weinberg, 2000).

At the beginning of the 21st century, six biological properties that cells developed when they became cancerous were proposed, called the hallmarks of cancer: maintenance of proliferative signaling, evasion of growth suppressive signals, invasion and metastasis activation, facilitation of replicative immortality, induction of angiogenesis and resistance to cell death. Subsequently, two emerging hallmarks were added: deregulation of cellular metabolism and immune system evasion, as well as two enabling characteristics: genomic instability and favoring inflammation (Hanahan & Weinberg, 2011).

However, certain errors in the regulation of the cell cycle are sufficient for the transformation of a normal cell into a cancer cell proliferation and excessive proliferation to occur. The cell cycle consists of four sequential phases: G1, S, G2, and M; the transition from one phase to another is very finely regulated by complex molecular mechanisms. The two main points that function as DNA damage sensors in which it is necessary to stop the cell cycle are G1/S and G2/M. Now, two proteins are widely involved in this fine regulation: retinoblastoma protein (pRB) and p53, also called the guardian of the genome. pRB can bind to the transcription factor E2F to prevent the G1/S transition and thus stop the cell cycle. p53 acts through p21 to regulate G1/S and G2M, can also induce BAX, an apoptosis gene, and thus contributes to cell cycle arrest, DNA repair, and apoptosis in the case of irreversible cell damage (Schafer, 1998).

The most classic example of malignant transformation by failures in cell cycle regulation can be seen in the etiopathogenesis of cervical cancer, in which the proteins of human papillomavirus E6 and E7 inhibit the activity of p53 and pRB, respectively, resulting in abnormal proliferation of damaged cells and, with it, the development of cancer (Szymonowicz & Chen, 2020).

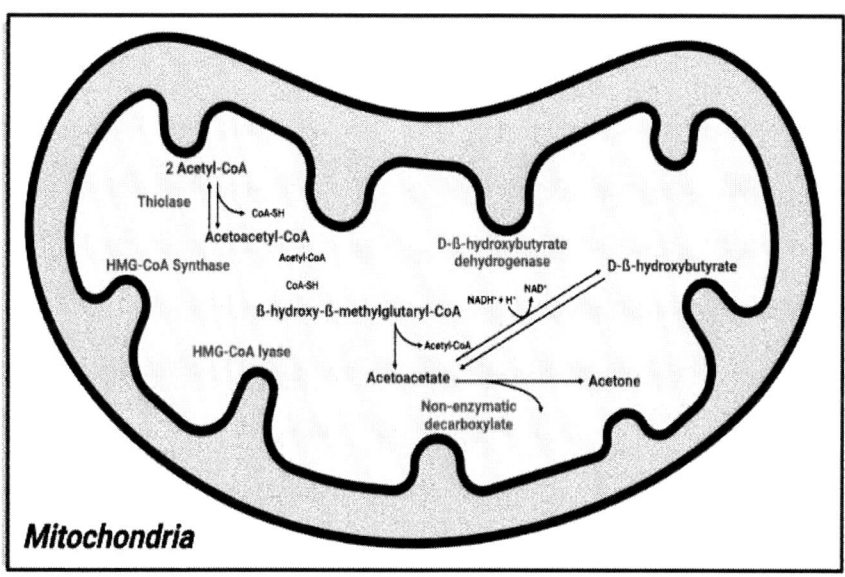

Figure 1. Ketogenesis. This process begins with the presence of a high rate of fatty acid oxidation in the liver, where mitochondria use acetyl-CoA from ß-oxidation to convert it to ketone bodies. In the first place, a thiolase inversion occurs where 2 moles of acetyl-CoA are converted to acetoacetyl-CoA, and later, acetoacetyl-CoA is converted to HMG-CoA via HMG-CoA. Finally, HMG-CoA under the action of HMG-CoA lyase produces AcAc and acetyl-CoA. AcAc undergoes a NADH-dependent reduction to give rise to D- BHB or, after spontaneous decarboxylation, produces acetone.

KD shares the main goal with other low-calorie diets such as prolonged fasting and caloric restriction and consists of maintaining safe ketosis levels through which ketone bodies induce molecular mechanisms that protect against certain diseases. Ketone bodies are produced mainly in the mitochondrial matrix of hepatocytes, although sometimes there may also be a small renal synthesis. First, an energy substrate provides two acetyl-CoA molecules to form acetoacetyl-CoA through the enzyme beta-ketothylase. Then, by the action of Hydroxymethylglutaril-CoA synthase (HMG-CoA) synthase, another molecule of acetyl-CoA condenses with acetoacetyl-CoA to form 3-hydroxy-3-methylglutaril-CoA. Later, it is hydrolyzed into an AcAc molecule and an acetyl-CoA molecule by the action of HMG-CoA lyase. Finally, some AcAc is reduced to BHB by BHB-dehydrogenase, while another part of AcAc undergoes spontaneous decarboxylation to transform into acetone. These three end products, AcAc, BHB and acetone, are molecules that possess biological activity related to the prevention and treatment of cancer (Puchalska & Crawford 2017; Ruan & Crawford 2018) (Figure 1).

It should be noted that AcAc and BHB are acids, so their excessive plasma levels can produce a decrease in blood pH, as occurs in diabetic ketoacidosis (Prisco et al., 2006). For this reason, KD-induced ketonemia in chronic diseases should be monitored at the time of induction to therapy.

Epigenetic Mechanisms

Epigenetics is responsible for studying gene expression and function changes, regardless of the DNA sequence itself. This is particularly important in cancer due to the expression of oncogenes, the signaling of cell differentiation, and sensitivity to radiation therapy and chemotherapy. The most representative epigenetic alterations can be grouped into changes in DNA methylation and histone modifications, in which diet and other environmental factors play a crucial role (Berger et al., 2009).

DNA methylation is a reaction in which methyl groups are added to DNA by methyltransferases, modifying their gene expression; thus, some cancer cells are able to deploy hypermethylation in the promoters' regions of tumor suppressor genes, achieving transcriptional silencing, as occurs in acute lymphoblastic leukemia secondary to mutations in the DNA methyltransferase 3 alpha gene (Bond et al., 2019). Nitrogenous DNA base pairs are wrapped and packaged under low molecular weight proteins called histones. This arrangement between DNA and histones is known as chromatin. When chromatin is dense and compact (heterochromatin), it is incapable of DNA transcription, while euchromatin is dispersed and transcriptionally active. This fine mechanism defines which genes will be expressed in each cell; however, histones may undergo modifications under chemical reactions of methylation, acetylation, and phosphorylation. Thus, MLL2 or KMT2D gene mutations, that encode a histone methyltransferase, are frequently found in follicular lymphoma (Morin et al., 2011).

The key step of KD in cancer prevention is post-translational histone modifications by ketone bodies. β-hydroxybutyrylation of lysine residues in histones can mediate gene expression and is present in vitro under ketonemia conditions. Furthermore, high concentrations of BHB inhibit class I deacetylase histones, and the acetylation of histones itself depends on blood levels of acetyl-CoA, which is directly related to liver generation of ketone bodies (Ruan & Crawford, 2018).

An alternate mechanism from which KD can act on cancer prevention is through non-coding RNAs. miR are small sequences of monocatenary RNA that regulate the translation of mRNA and thus control cell growth and differentiation. Onco-miR and miR tumor suppressors have been identified. The mi-RNA 21 gene is elevated in neoplasms such as hepatocellular carcinoma and multiple myeloma, which could be a target for ketone bodies. A recent study found an association in the expression of miR secondary to KD in humans; epigenetic changes of KD in cancer prevention were evidenced in miR-504-5p, which is related to the genes TP53, VEGFA, MDM2, TFF1, TCEA1 and DRD1 (Cannataro et al., 2019).

The usefulness of KD through these epigenetic therapeutic targets has already been demonstrated in animal models of gliomas, as well as prostate cancer and digestive tract cancers.

Energy Metabolism

Energy metabolism homeostasis in any organism is essential to maintaining proper cellular function. Anything that modifies basal metabolism, such as a KD or cancer development, has the capacity to affect cellular communication, differentiation, and gene transcription positively or negatively (Barry et al., 2018).

When we talk about KD, we are not referring to just one type of diet, as there are variations of it, either through caloric restriction, intermittent fasting, or simply an average caloric intake with a higher percentage of fats (Barzegar et al., 2021). Standard KDs are characterized by containing four parts of fat (in the form of long chains) and one part of proteins and carbohydrates, supplemented with minerals and vitamins (O'Neill & Raggi, 2020). In the end, KD, whatever its variant, seeks the same thing: to manipulate the energy metabolism in our favor. Let us remember that metabolism under physiological conditions work on our most important substrate, glucose. In situations where glucose cannot meet the energy demand, biochemical mechanisms such as ketogenesis are activated as an alternative source to produce substrates that maintain cellular functioning.

The state of ketonemia induced by KD is obtained by the production of ketone bodies (acetone, AcAc and BHB) from fatty acids within the mitochondria of hepatocytes, a process called ketogenesis. The lipid substrate will enter the β-oxidation pathway to be converted to acetyl CoA, which the target cell will use to initiate the Krebs cycle (Dhillon & Gupta, 2022). Of the three ketone bodies produced, AcAc and BHB are the ones used by tissues to produce energy. Thus, BHB is released into the portal circulation and, when it reaches the extrahepatic tissue, it is converted to AcAc by the enzyme BHB dehydrogenase. AcAc will then be used through the ketolysis pathway to convert back to acetyl CoA by the enzyme β-ketoacyl-CoA transferase (Newman & Verdin, 2017). After oxidative phosphorylation of acetyl-CoA, 22 adenosine triphosphate (ATP) molecules will be produced (compared to 38 ATP molecules produced through glycolysis).

One of the hallmarks of tumor cells is their ability to modify or reprogram their energy metabolism. A cancer cell is characterized by chronic, uncontrolled, and accelerated proliferation, a process that requires a large amount of energy, so it will do everything in its power to have the necessary fuel to cope with its growth and division. Under normal conditions, glucose oxidation in cells depends on the oxygen concentration in the microenvironment (Figure 2). In an aerobic condition, cells first use glycolysis to produce pyruvate and then deliver it to the mitochondria, forming carbon dioxide. In anaerobconditions, glycolysis is favored, sending little pyruvate to the mitochondria. In the context of neoplastic cells, they can reprogram glucose oxidation so that in the absence or presence of oxygen, they will limit energy metabolism to a greater extent toward glycolysis (Figure 2). This is known as aerobic glycolysis or Warburg effect (Hanahan & Weinberg, 2011).

The preference towards the glycolytic pathway will ultimately be carried out by the overregulation of glucose transporters, especially GLUT1, which promotes increased glucose uptake and, thus, glucose utilization. The glycolytic dependence of tumor cells may even be accentuated under hypoxic conditions, as it is characteristic of many tumors, where mechanisms triggered in response to hypoxia overregulate enzymes of the glycolytic pathway and glucose transporters through upregulation of transcription factors such as HIF1α and HIF2α. The aforementioned has also been linked to activated oncogenes (such as RAS) and mutant tumor suppressors, allow for other tumor cell hallmarks such as attenuation of apoptosis, evasion of cytokine control, or cell proliferation.

The Warburg effect may not seem physiologically desirable, since cancer cells must compensate for the 18-fold lower efficiency of ATP molecule production offered by glycolysis compared to that offered by oxidative phosphorylation in mitochondria (Bose & Le, 2018). Ultimately, this increase in the glycolytic pathway will allow the diversion of glycolytic intermediates to biosynthesis pathways to generate nucleotides or amino acids, allowing in turn the synthesis of organelles and macromolecules necessary for the assembly of new cells (note how this metabolic switch favors the unregulated division characteristic of tumor cells).

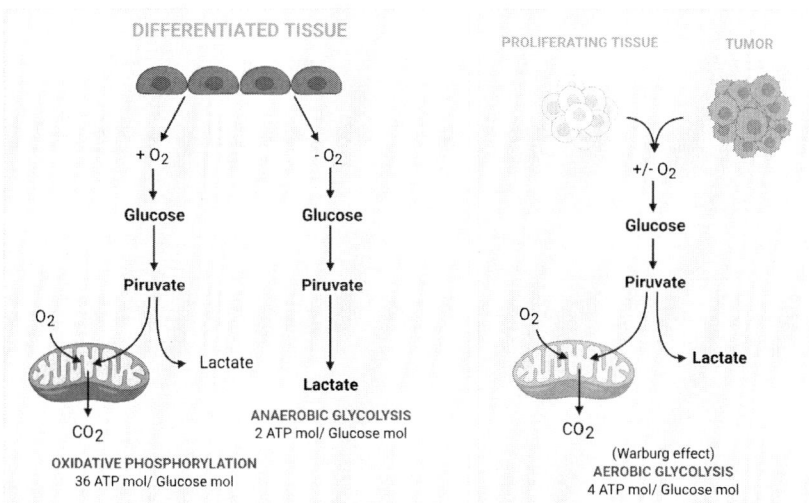

Figure 2. Under normal conditions, cells produce ATP to meet the needs through two mechanisms: glycolysis and the Krebs cycle. The end product can be lactate or, upon complete glucose oxidation through respiration in the mitochondria, CO_2. In tumors and other proliferating cells, the rate of glucose uptake dramatically increases, and lactate is produced, even in the presence of oxygen and fully functioning mitochondria. This is known as aerobic glycolysis or the Warburg effect.

The tumor microenvironment can become more complex as it has been seen that in some cancer cell subpopulations, there are differences between energy production pathways. Here, the metabolism of one cell subgroup will be glucose dependent (through the Warburg effect) and will produce lactate. This lactate will then be taken up by the second neighboring cell subgroup and used as its main energy source through the tricarboxylic acid cycle (TCA) pathway (Kennedy & Dewhirst, 2010). This mechanism is essential in the neoplastic cell, since unstable tumor-associated neovascularization causes a disorganization of the local oxygen supply. Intratumoral symbiosis will allow cells in a more hypoxic environment to rely mainly on glucose, producing lactate as a waste product that will be used by better-oxygenated cells.

One of the adjuvant or nonpharmacological measures that has been proposed in the treatment of cancer is precisely KD, which has several antitumor mechanisms. KD, as previously mentioned, consists of reducing the intake of carbohydrates, especially in the caloric restriction variant. This will cause blood glucose concentrations to decrease and, therefore, the tumor cell will be induced to chronic metabolic stress because it will not have its main substrate to perform aerobic glycolysis (Weber et al., 2020). Similarly, the reduction in glucose will be accompanied by a reduction in circulating levels of insulin and insulin-like growth factor. Both are known to activate signaling pathways through their receptors and contribute to tumorigenesis. Mutations of the insulin-activated enzyme gene of phosphatidylinositol 3-kinase (PI3K) are known in tumors, demonstrating enhanced activity. For this reason, there is a group of drugs that act as inhibitors of this enzyme, however, it has been seen that as a side effect, by inhibiting the enzyme, these drugs cause reactive hyperglycemia that leads to an increase in insulin levels, and this in turn reactivates the PI3K pathway in the form of resistance to treatment. The KD can help to enhance the effect of these inhibitors, as it limits this glucose-insulin feedback system, blocking its reactivation (Drullinsky & Hurvitz, 2020). Another KD effect includes the decrease in lactic acid concentrations in tumor tissue. Lactic acid serves as a product of aerobic glycolysis and therefore accumulates in most cancer cells, allowing its utilization as fuel (Weber et al., 2018).

KD not only has the ability to affect tumor glucose metabolism, but also can affect mitochondrial metabolism. Cancer is ultimately a mitochondrial disease, as cancer cells fail in their cellular respiration processes due to an alteration at the mitochondrial oxidative phosphorylation system (OXPHOS) level. This can be due to different reasons, from mutations in the genes encoding the OXPHOS system, reduction of this complex, or reduced mitochondrial mass. Tumor cells to compensate for their energy requirements affected by mitochondrial dysfunction use aerobic fermentation. When KD induces a state of ketosis, it is necessary for the tumor to have functional mitochondria to use ketone bodies and survive, so tumor cells lacking this feature are subjected to high metabolic stress (Luo et al., 2020). KD can not only modify the course of metabolism in tumors with mitochondrial dysfunction. Rapidly growing tumors develop hypoxic areas, so in the context of a ketonic state, for the cancer cell to take advantage of ketone bodies, there must be an adequate concentration of oxygen. Therefore, even if the tumor cell has functional mitochondria, diet-induced ketosis makes the cell incapable of producing energy (Srinivasan et al., 2017). It is also important to mention that the degree of impact of KD will depend on practically three mitochondrial enzymes (BDH1, SCOT, and ACAT1) and how functional they are in the tumor cell, since these enzymes will allow it to degrade ketones to produce energy.

Finally, KD also plays a role in modifying amino acid metabolism and urea cycle metabolites in tumor cells. There has been seen that there exists an alteration in the metabolism of amino acids such as serine, glycine, tryptophan, or glutamate-glutamine, proposing that the KD leads to a down-regulation of amino acid-dependent metabolic processes to conserve them (Weber, 2020). This is important because a large group of tumors depend on the metabolism of amino acids such as glutamate-glutamine. It seems that KD with a low protein intake induces a lack of the essential amino acids the tumor cell needs, thus inhibiting its growth (Vettore et al., 2020).

Anti-Inflammatory Mechanisms

Inflammation constitutes a crucial component of the innate immune system's reaction to tissue damage or infection, playing a pivotal role in the mobilization of circulating cells and antibodies that contribute to the adaptive immunological response within the affected tissue (Coussens & Werb, 2002). The process is initiated by resident cells within the tissue, which possess the ability to detect pathogens or injuries. These cells then transmit alarm signals in the form of chemical messengers, thereby enhancing the local response and attracting additional cells to the affected region. According to Pahwa et al. (2022), the presence of chronic inflammation has the potential to facilitate the development of cancer, whereas inflammation caused by tumors can sustain the advancement of tumors. According to estimates, a significant proportion of cancer cases, up to 20%, can be attributed to the presence of chronic inflammation or persistent infections.

Inflammatory cytokines and cells have been identified as key factors in developing and advancing tumors in several locations, including the stomach, colon, skin, liver, breast, lung, and head/neck. Extensive research has provided substantial evidence supporting their involvement in carcinogenesis and tumor progression in these specific cancer types. Several significant routes have been found connecting inflammation with the initiation or progression of tumors. The presence of an inflammatory environment is characterized by increased concentrations of nuclear factor κB (NF-κB), reactive oxygen and nitrogen species, cytokines, prostaglandins, and miR. These molecular factors have significant impacts on several cellular processes, including cell proliferation, cell death, cell senescence, DNA mutation rates, DNA methylation, and angiogenesis (Murata, 2018).

Cytokines, including IL-6, are observed in numerous types of cancer and have been associated with the development of tumors and the spread of cancer cells by modulating the activity of NF-κB and STAT3 signaling pathways. The correlation between inflammation and cancer is widely supported by scientific evidence, particularly within the digestive system. In this context, inflammation arises from several factors, such as dietary choices, the gut microbiota, infections, or autoimmune conditions, that are frequently observed. Chronic ulcerative colitis and Crohn's disease have been found to increase the likelihood of developing colon cancer. Similarly, acid reflux has been associated with the appearance of esophageal cancer. Furthermore, hepatitis C infection and alcohol consumption have been identified as factors that increase the risk of hepatocellular carcinoma. Additionally, the presence of Helicobacter pylori infection has been associated with increased susceptibility to gastric and colon cancer (Mundi et al., 2021).

Chronic inflammation that occurs before carcinogenesis shares certain characteristics with the acute physiological process. Certain types of food have the potential to contribute to the development of chronic inflammation, which, in turn, can facilitate the occurrence of gastrointestinal malignancies. Although the precise mechanisms underlying the connection between nutrition and inflammation remain incompletely elucidated, certain instances have firmly proven this relationship (Singh et al., 2019). The long-term use of alcohol induces mast cell activation, leading to polyp development and promotion of tumor growth and invasion in a mouse model of colon cancer. Certain instances have revealed the identification of particular antigens that possess the ability to trigger and perpetuate the inflammatory process. For example, research has shown that red meat is characterized by elevated concentrations of N-glycolylneuraminic acid, a type of sialic acid that is not naturally produced by humans. The introduction of this exogenous antigen has the potential to be assimilated into the surrounding tissue, thereby eliciting the recruitment of inflammatory cells. Obesity-related malignancies have been found to have a connection with inflammation. The increasing global incidence of obesity has generated significant academic attention to understand the increased susceptibility to cancer among people who are overweight or obese (Wright & Simone, 2016). A significant portion of research efforts are directed towards investigating the role of obesity-caused inflammation, as it has been established that such inflammation is associated with the progression of cancer at multiple locations. In the presence of chronic inflammation, the bloodstream contains cytokines and other associated substances.

Inflammation is one of the most important hallmarks of cancer development and its progression. There is a direct connection between inflammation and tumorigenesis, including proliferation, invasion, angiogenesis, and metastasis (Mantovani et al., 2008). The NOD-like receptor pyrin domain containing 3 inflammasome (NLRP3) plays an important role in this inflammatory response. The NLRP3 inflammasome is a multimeric protein complex that assembles in response to cellular perturbations (Moossavi et al., 2018).

An inflammasome is a multimolecular complex, composed of a NOD-like protein (NLR), the adaptor-associated apoptosis-associated speck-like protein containing a caspase recruitment domain (ASC), and caspase-1, which is responsible for the cleavage of pro-IL-1β and pro-IL-8 proteins in their active forms. Therefore, the production of mature or active IL-1β is controlled by at least two molecular mechanisms: first, Toll-like receptor (TLR) ligands or endogenous danger signals induce the expression of pro-IL-1β mRNA and proteins; the second signal triggered by very diverse stimuli activates inflammasomes, leading to IL-1β maturation and secretion of IL-1. The NOD-like receptor family, NLRP3, is the most studied in this group, but other inflammasomes, including NLRP1, NLRC4, and absent in the inflammasomes of melanoma 2ASC, have also been identified. Although many stimuli with very different and unrelated molecular structures induce activation of the NLRP3 inflammasome, the signal mechanisms that lead to the activation of the inflammasome remain elusive. This assembly allows the activation of caspase-1, which promotes the release of the inflammatory cytokines interleukin-1β (IL-1β) and IL-18, as well as inflammatory cell death (pyroptosis). Inflammatory cytokines contribute to the development of low-grade systemic inflammation, and aberrant activation of NLRP3 can drive a chronic inflammatory state in the body to modulate the pathogenesis of diseases associated with inflammation (Moossavi et al., 2018). Therefore, fine-tuning the activity of the NLRP3 inflammasome is essential to maintain proper cellular homeostasis and health. Here, we will cover the mechanisms of activation of the NLRP3 inflammasome and its divergent roles in the pathogenesis of inflammation-associated diseases such as cancer, atherosclerosis, diabetes, and obesity, highlighting the therapeutic potential of targeting this pathway (Figure 3).

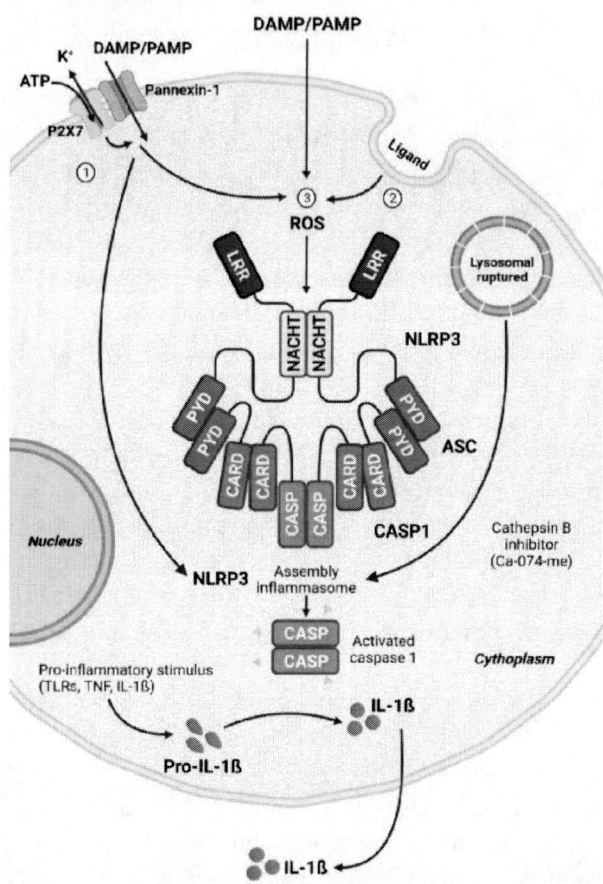

Figure 3. The NLRP3 inflammasome is a critical component of the innate immune system that mediates caspase-1 activation and the secretion of pro-inflammatory cytokines in response to cellular damage. The priming step is induced by TLRs and cytokine receptors, such as the tumor necrosis factor (TNF) receptor or IL-1 receptor (IL-1R), which recognize pathogen-associated molecular patterns (PAMPs) or Damage-associated molecular patterns (DAMPs) and upregulate the transcription of NLRP3 and IL1β. PAMPs and DAMPs then promote NLRP3 inflammasome assembly, thereby leading to caspase 1-mediated inflammatory cytokine maturation and release, and pyroptosis.

NLRP3 can have opposing roles in tumorigenesis. It can be tumor-suppressive, which has mainly been shown in the context of colitis-associated colorectal cancer. Still, it can also be tumor-promoting, with these effects being more evident in other forms of cancer, such as gastric and skin cancer (Mundi et al., 2021).

Cancer exhibits an altered metabolism compared to normal cells. It has been shown that cancer cells can increase the rate of glycolytic metabolism to support increased cancer cell proliferation and energy demands, even in the presence of oxygen with excessive lactate production (Warburg effect) (Allen et al., 2014). Increased glucose metabolism promotes excessive proliferation, antiapoptotic signaling, cell cycle progression, and angiogenesis. Defects of glycolytic and ketolytic enzymes in the mitochondria of tumor cells explain the preference for glycolysis instead of oxidative phosphorylation to produce ATP. Cancer cells show higher levels of steady-state oxidative stress than normal cells, making them more sensitive to apoptotic stimuli mediated by reactive oxygen species. Also, the microenvironment is acidified, which promotes metastasis (Barrea et al., 2022).

Systemic inflammation is a central and reversible mechanism through which obesity promotes tumor risk and progression. Patients with obesity have inflamed adipose tissue, with immune cell infiltration and remodeling. This local inflamed environment is related to different pathophysiologic modifications that may promote a variety of cancers. In systemic inflammation, other metabolic diseases may occur, including metabolic syndrome and insulin resistance, that operate in concert with local mechanisms of cancer to increase the inflammatory state and promote tumor growth and progression (Kuchkuntla et al., 2019).

Although systemic glucose is limited, normal tissues will shift cellular energy supply from glucose to fatty acid and ketones to protect against hypoglycemia. Ketone bodies may increase oxidative stress in cancer cells by entering the TCA cycle due to abnormalities in mitochondrial structure and function.

Ketone bodies serve as an alternative energy source to glucose fasting, they are mainly produced during fasting and prolonged or intense physical activity. Ketone bodies are transported in the blood to tissues where they are converted to acetyl-CoA, a substrate in the first step of the citric acid cycle to obtain energy (Feng et al., 2019).

Ketone metabolism results in a decreased production of reactive oxygen species, which is known to contribute to inflammation. Adenosine acting through A1 and A2 receptor subtypes limits inflammation in various peripheral and central tissues, including inflammation due to subcutaneous inflammogens. Polyunsaturated fatty acid-induced activation of PPAR inhibits NFκB and AP-1, both pro-inflammatory transcription factors. It is possible that each is involved, and more research is needed to elucidate the primary mechanism underlying this peripheral effect. In addition to specific cellular mechanisms, protein restriction reduces inflammation in some situations, and caloric restriction is generally anti-inflammatory.

Anticarcinogenic effects of KD implicate that mitochondrial dysfunction of cancer cells, and concomitantly reduced expression of ketolytic enzymes, may contribute to this effect (Zhu et al., 2022). When blood glucose levels drop, cancer cells starve, while normal cells change their metabolism to utilize ketone bodies to survive. Furthermore, the decrease in insulin level that accompanies the indicated ketonemic conditions correlates with a decrease in insulin-like growth factors, which promotes the proliferation of cancer cells.

The currently available medical literature provides evidence for the safe application of a KD only in patients with glioblastoma. However, some promising evidence in favor of KD has also been reported in the treatment of prostate, colon, pancreas, and lung cancers. On the contrary, only limited evidence is available on the anticancer effect of KD on stomach and liver cancer.

Cancer Treatment

Hippocrates believed that food plays an important role in health expressing it with the phrase "Let food be thy medicine and medicine be thy food" (Mittelman, 2020).

The effect of KD as an adjuvant in the treatment of cancer has been studied, the traditional KD consists of a 4:1 ratio of fat to protein plus carbohydrates, with this diet providing 90% of calories, 8% protein, and 2% carbohydrates (deCampo & Kossoff., 2019), finding beneficial effects to improve the quality of life of patients, in addition to causing little or no added toxicity (Zhu et al., 2022; Weber et al., 2020). Some studies show that this type of diet is well tolerated by patients under chemotherapy. In addition to helping reduce their fatigue after chemotherapies (Tan-Shalaby, 2017). With the application of the KD, cancer cells have less glucose; therefore, they cannot use ketone bodies as a source of energy because of abnormal mitochondrial function and decreased enzymatic activity for the use of ketones. At the same time, it could affect glucose metabolism and glucose-dependent signaling in cancer cells, as a consequence of glucose depletion in aberrant cells, there is a cessation of lactate/pyruvate cycling, stopping epidermal necrosis factor, neovascularization, and angiogenesis, causing necrosis in tumor cells (Weber et al., 2020).

KD is also known to cause inhibition of the NLRP3 inflammasome, resulting in a stroke.

Decreased inflammation by BHB, which is helpful since inflammation is related in the pathophysiology of cancer. It also acts by stopping cancer cell transcription and proliferation (Tan-Shalaby, 2017).

Tests have been performed in mouse cancer models in which it has been obtained that this type of diet has positive effects on anti-PI3K treatment (phosphatidylinisitol 3-kinase inhibitors) since the use of these drugs alone causes hyperglycemia by increasing insulin levels and activating the PI3K pathway, which is commonly activated by human malignant tumors, plus, it is usually genetically mutated in some cancers (Talib et al., 2021) with the implementation of this diet the acute glucose-insulin cycle is suppressed demonstrating that the KD is a good adjuvant with pharmacological therapy (Weber et al., 2020). In addition, it has been found in mouse models of metastatic cancer that exogenous ketone can have cytotoxic effects on tumor proliferation. (Tan-Shalaby, 2017).

Other benefits are the decrease of hyperglycemia and insulin secretion (Weber et al., 2020). and at the same time, it can cause a decrease in the intratumoral mTorc1 signaling pathway, which is part of the target of the rapamycin (TOR) family of proteins, they are involved in the regulation of mRNA transcription and protein translation, in addition to being involved in maintaining proper functioning of signaling pathways and cell cycle succession. The mTORc1 pathway is one of the complexes of the TOR protein family, this complex is sensitive to rapamycin and has the raptor protein, there is a second complex called mTORC2 which has the Rictor protein (Sarbassov et al., 2005).

It is discussed that KD and its effect, whether beneficial or not, depends on the type or subtype of cancer, as well as genetic background; therefore, it should be studied thoroughly before recommending therapy to all cancer patients (Weber et al., 2018).

Among the studies that have been conducted to determine the effects of KD as a therapy in cancer, results have been obtained, among which stand out that KD has beneficial effects in the prevention of tumors, it has also been documented that it can delay tumor growth (Otto et al., 2008) and even delays the onset of cachexia that occurs in people with cancer, (Weber et al., 2020) it has also been documented that it can increase the survival of people with this pathology in addition to being able to sensitize the tumor cells to have a better adjuvant effect in chemotherapy or radiation therapy. There are studies of cases of neuroblastoma in which KD can stop its growth (Weber et al., 2020).

Practically, three variables can be obtained as a result of the implementation of this diet: having an antitumor effect and helping to improve the quality of life of patients, having adverse effects although in clinical trials there are no records of serious adverse effects, or having no significant effect on tumor growth (Weber et al., 2020).

Some of the reports described in recent articles documented the case of 2 pediatric female patients with malignant astrocytoma already in the advanced stages of the disease, KD was introduced into the diet of both children for 2 months, imaging studies were performed, it was documented that 7 days after the implementation of the diet, blood glucose levels decreased while ketone bodies were elevated and an improvement in mood and quality of life was observed (Nebeling et al., 1995).

The positive effects of the implementation of this diet are that it can help maintain lipid profiles in balance in cancer patients. The mechanisms by which it can act in the treatment of cancer are due to the antitumor effects of AcAc and BHB ketone bodies due to their antiproliferative effect (Weber et al., 2020). This type of diet generates a chronic metabolic stress effect that intervenes in the Warburg effect of cancer cells that affect tumor proliferation (Tan-Shalaby, 2017). It has also been reported that there can be a marked decrease in glucose in conjunction with caloric restriction, as it has shown favorable results in preventing tumor growth (Tan-Shalaby, 2017).

The KD has a great impact on the mitochondria of cancer cells, some tumors have a reduction in the mass of their mitochondria or a reduction in one or more of the OXPHOS complexes (Tan-Shalaby, 2017) depending on the type of cancer; therefore, cancer; therefore, these tumors must use anaerobic fermentation, the KD generates significant metabolic stress in tumors that have dysfunctional mitochondria or have a low amount of mitochondria, there are 3 mitochondrial enzymes that are SCOT, ACAT1, BDH1, these are important for the utilization of ketone bodies and the functionality of the KD. Rodent studies have shown that KD can influence amino acid metabolism and urea cycle metabolites. There are in vitro studies showing that KD and ketogenic bodies cause an anti-inflammatory effect by suppressing the NLRP3 inflammasome, interleukins such as 1-6 and prostaglandin E2 (Weber et al., 2020).

The influence of KD on gene expression has been described, as it is able to modulate gene expression. The prolonged use of KD has had an effect on stabilizing lysine acetylation and p53 helping to prevent cancer in mice, p53 is a tumor suppressor responsible for controlling processes such as apoptosis and genetic stability (Talib et al., 2021).

Experimental studies were carried out at the University of Lowa in which KD was applied together with radiation therapy and chemotherapy in mice containing MIA PaCa 2 pancreatic cancer xenografts and in mice with non-small cell lung cancer, fractionated radiation (2 Gy / fx) was performed to measure tumor growth and 4-hydroxy-2-nonenal was used as an oxidative stress marker to look for modified proteins; the results obtained indicated that mice with pancreatic cancer xenografts with KD and radiation therapy had longer survival compared to those treated with radiation therapy alone. As for mice with non-small cell lung cancer, they did not have adequate control of KD and therefore did not have optimal results (Zahra et al., 2017).

Table 1. Studies that have assessed the effects of the KD on cancer

Author, year	Study Design	Sample size	Outcomes
Maurer et al., (2011).	Role of KD in tumor cell energy metabolism in rat hippocampal neurons and 5 glioma cell lines. A KD was examined in an orthotopic xenograft glioma mouse model.	Total: 24 female mice. Randomly divided into 2 groups. Group 1: Carbohydrate rich diet vs. Group 2: KD.	The KD increased blood BHB. There were no alterations in blood glucose levels. No improvement in survival.
Otto et al., (2008).	The mouse xenograft model was used. They were injected subcutaneously with tumor cells of the gastric adenocarcinoma cell line 23132/87. The two diets were compared according to tumor growth and survival time.	Total: 24 female mice. They were divided into 2 groups: KD group: 12 SD group: 12	In the KD group: Adequate acceptance of KD. Delayed tumor growth compared to the SD group.
Nebeling et al., (1995).	To confirm whether KD can decrease glucose availability in some tumors.	Total: 2 female pediatrics. Patients with advanced stage malignant	Decreased blood glucosa levels

Table 1. (Continued)

Author, year	Study Design	Sample size	Outcomes
Schmidt et al., (2011).	Prospective, observational pilot study. The aim was to investigate whether DK is safe, without adverse effects in patients with advanced cancer and without therapeutic options.	Total: 16 patients with advanced metastatic tumors. 2 groups: n = 13 DK > 3 weeks. n = 3 without DK.	KD can decrease classical blood parameters. Weight Loss in participants. Improvement in quality of life.
Kasumi and Sato, (2019).	Implementing KD in a mouse model with peritoneal dissemination. BALB/c mice were inoculated intraperitoneally with colon 26, a murine colon adenocarcinoma cell line, to induce experimental peritoneal dissemination.	Male, 5-week-old BALB/c mice. 2 groups: Group with KD. Group without KD.	Improved survival in KD mice and better health status with KD. KD as preventive therapy for peritoneal dissemination. Tumor weight was not significantly lower in the KD group.

The implementation of KD in experimental studies and in humans with malignant tumors can be considered favorable in conjunction with conventional treatments such as radiotherapy, chemotherapy, or surgical treatment, although there is still a long way to explore in this area and in the development of more studies in humans and in experimental animals, as well as in various types of cancer, in order to obtain a greater number of results, we believe that the KD has a favorable future in the adjuvant treatment of cancer as well as for its prevention.

Conclusion

The KD has enough evidence to be a great ally in the prevention and treatment of cancer. Some of the mechanisms by which it is reasonable that ketone bodies have antiproliferative properties are already known; however, it is necessary to follow strict medical recommendations to avoid the adverse effects that ketosis could cause. Likewise, KD is a turning point for the incursion of more dietary modifications as an aid in the management of chronic diseases. It is necessary to continue extensive cancer research, a disease that, despite the development of technology, is becoming more prevalent around the world.

Disclaimer

None.

Acknowledgments

We thank the Armstrong Foundation for the undergraduate scholarship to David Vazquez.

References

Allen, B. G., Bhatia, S. K., Anderson, C. M., Eichenberger-Gilmore, J. M., Sibenaller, Z. A., Mapuskar, K. A., Schoenfeld, J. D., Buatti, J. M., Spitz, D. R., & Fath, M. A. (2014). Ketogenic diets as an adjuvant cancer therapy: History and potential mechanism. *Redox Biology*, *2*, 963–970. https://doi.org/10.1016/j.redox.2014.08.002

Anna Szymonowicz, K., & Chen, J. (2020). Biological and clinical aspects of HPV-related cancers. *Cancer Biology and Medicine*, *17*(4), 864–878. https://doi.org/10.20892/j.issn.2095-3941.2020.0370

Barrea, L., Caprio, M., Tuccinardi, D., Moriconi, E., Di Renzo, L., Muscogiuri, G., Colao, A., & Savastano, S. (2022). Could ketogenic diet "starve" cancer? Emerging evidence. *Critical Reviews in Food Science and Nutrition*, *62*(7), 1800–1821. https://doi.org/10.1080/10408398.2020.1847030

Barry, D., Ellul, S., Watters, L., Lee, D., Haluska, R., & White, R. (2018). The ketogenic diet in disease and development. *International Journal of Developmental Neuroscience*, *68*(1), 53–58. https://doi.org/10.1016/j.ijdevneu.2018.04.005

Barzegar, M., Afghan, M., Tarmahi, V., Behtari, M., Rahimi Khamaneh, S., & Raeisi, S. (2021). Ketogenic diet: overview, types, and possible anti-seizure mechanisms. *Nutritional Neuroscience*, *24*(4), 307–316. https://doi.org/10.1080/1028415X.2019.1627769

Berger, S. L., Kouzarides, T., Shiekhattar, R., & Shilatifard, A. (2009). An operational definition of epigenetics: Figure 1. *Genes & Development*, *23*(7), 781–783. https://doi.org/10.1101/gad.1787609

Bond, J., Touzart, A., Leprêtre, S., Graux, C., Bargetzi, M., Lhermitte, L., Hypolite, G., Leguay, T., Hicheri, Y., Guillerm, G., Bilger, K., Lhéritier, V., Hunault, M., Huguet,

F., Chalandon, Y., Ifrah, N., Macintyre, E., Dombret, H., Asnafi, V., & Boissel, N. (2019). *DNMT3A*mutation is associated with increased age and adverse outcome in adult T-cell acute lymphoblastic leukemia. *Haematologica*, *104*(8), 1617–1625. https://doi.org/10.3324/haematol.2018.197848

Bose, S., & Le, A. (2018). *Glucose Metabolism in Cancer* (pp. 3–12). https://doi.org/10.1007/978-3-319-77736-8_1

Cannataro, R., Perri, M., Gallelli, L., Caroleo, M. C., De Sarro, G., & Cione, E. (2019). Ketogenic Diet Acts on Body Remodeling and MicroRNAs Expression Profile. *MicroRNA*, *8*(2), 116–126. https://doi.org/10.2174/2211536608666181126093903

Coussens, L. M., & Werb, Z. (2002). Inflammation and cancer. *Nature*, *420*(6917), 860–867. https://doi.org/10.1038/nature01322

deCampo, D. M., & Kossoff, E. H. (2019). Ketogenic dietary therapies for epilepsy and beyond. *Current Opinion in Clinical Nutrition & Metabolic Care*, *22*(4), 264–268. https://doi.org/10.1097/MCO.0000000000000565

Dhillon, K. K., & Gupta, S. (2024). *Biochemistry, Ketogenesis*.

Dowis, K., & Banga, S. (2021). The Potential Health Benefits of the Ketogenic Diet: A Narrative Review. *Nutrients*, *13*(5), 1654. https://doi.org/10.3390/nu13051654

Drullinsky, P. R., & Hurvitz, S. A. (2020). Mechanistic basis for PI3K inhibitor antitumor activity and adverse reactions in advanced breast cancer. *Breast Cancer Research and Treatment*, *181*(2), 233–248. https://doi.org/10.1007/s10549-020-05618-1

Feng, S., Wang, H., Liu, J., AA, J., Zhou, F., & Wang, G. (2019). Multi-dimensional roles of ketone bodies in cancer biology: Opportunities for cancer therapy. *Pharmacological Research*, *150*, 104500. https://doi.org/10.1016/j.phrs.2019.104500

Hajdu, S. I. (2011). A note from history: Landmarks in history of cancer, part 1. *Cancer*, *117*(5), 1097–1102. https://doi.org/10.1002/cncr.25553

Hanahan, D., & Weinberg, R. A. (2000). The Hallmarks of Cancer. *Cell*, *100*(1), 57–70. https://doi.org/10.1016/S0092-8674(00)81683-9

Hanahan, D., & Weinberg, R. A. (2011). Hallmarks of Cancer: The Next Generation. *Cell*, *144*(5), 646–674. https://doi.org/10.1016/j.cell.2011.02.013

Kennedy, K. M., & Dewhirst, M. W. (2010). Tumor metabolism of lactate: the influence and therapeutic potential for MCT and CD147 regulation. *Future Oncology*, *6*(1), 127–148. https://doi.org/10.2217/fon.09.145

Kuchkuntla, A. R., Shah, M., Velapati, S., Gershuni, V. M., Rajjo, T., Nanda, S., Hurt, R. T., & Mundi, M. S. (2019). Ketogenic Diet: an Endocrinologist Perspective. *Current Nutrition Reports*, *8*(4), 402–410. https://doi.org/10.1007/s13668-019-00297-x

Luo, Y., Ma, J., & Lu, W. (2020). The Significance of Mitochondrial Dysfunction in Cancer. *International Journal of Molecular Sciences*, *21*(16), 5598. https://doi.org/10.3390/ijms21165598

Mantovani, A., Allavena, P., Sica, A., & Balkwill, F. (2008). Cancer-related inflammation. *Nature*, *454*(7203), 436–444. https://doi.org/10.1038/nature07205

Mittelman, S. D. (2020). The Role of Diet in Cancer Prevention and Chemotherapy Efficacy. *Annual Review of Nutrition*, *40*(1), 273–297. https://doi.org/10.1146/annurev-nutr-013120-041149

Moossavi, M., Parsamanesh, N., Bahrami, A., Atkin, S. L., & Sahebkar, A. (2018). Role of the NLRP3 inflammasome in cancer. *Molecular Cancer*, *17*(1), 158. https://doi.org/10.1186/s12943-018-0900-3

Morin, R. D., Mendez-Lago, M., Mungall, A. J., Goya, R., Mungall, K. L., Corbett, R. D., Johnson, N. A., Severson, T. M., Chiu, R., Field, M., Jackman, S., Krzywinski, M., Scott, D. W., Trinh, D. L., Tamura-Wells, J., Li, S., Firme, M. R., Rogic, S., Griffith, M., … Marra, M. A. (2011). Frequent mutation of histone-modifying genes in non-Hodgkin lymphoma. *Nature*, *476*(7360), 298–303. https://doi.org/10.1038/nature10351

Mundi, M. S., Mohamed Elfadil, O., Patel, I., Patel, J., & Hurt, R. T. (2021). Ketogenic diet and cancer: Fad or fabulous? *Journal of Parenteral and Enteral Nutrition*, *45*(S2). https://doi.org/10.1002/jpen.2226

Murata, M. (2018). Inflammation and cancer. *Environmental Health and Preventive Medicine*, *23*(1), 50. https://doi.org/10.1186/s12199-018-0740-1

Nebeling, L. C., Miraldi, F., Shurin, S. B., & Lerner, E. (1995). Effects of a ketogenic diet on tumor metabolism and nutritional status in pediatric oncology patients: two case reports. *Journal of the American College of Nutrition*, *14*(2), 202–208. https://doi.org/10.1080/07315724.1995.10718495

Newman, J. C., & Verdin, E. (2017). β-Hydroxybutyrate: A Signaling Metabolite. *Annual Review of Nutrition*, *37*(1), 51–76. https://doi.org/10.1146/annurev-nutr-071816-064916

O'Neill, B., & Raggi, P. (2020). The ketogenic diet: Pros and cons. *Atherosclerosis*, *292*, 119–126. https://doi.org/10.1016/j.atherosclerosis.2019.11.021

Otto, C., Kaemmerer, U., Illert, B., Muehling, B., Pfetzer, N., Wittig, R., Voelker, H. U., Thiede, A., & Coy, J. F. (2008). Growth of human gastric cancer cells in nude mice is delayed by a ketogenic diet supplemented with omega-3 fatty acids and medium-chain triglycerides. *BMC Cancer*, *8*(1), 122. https://doi.org/10.1186/1471-2407-8-122

Pahwa, R., Goyal, A., & Jialal, I. (2024). *Chronic Inflammation*.

Prisco, F., Picardi, A., Iafusco, D., Lorini, R., Minicucci, L., Martinucci, M. E., Toni, S., Cerutti, F., Rabbone, I., Buzzetti, R., Crino, A., & Pozzilli, P. (2006). Blood ketone bodies in patients with recent-onset type 1 diabetes (a multicenter study). *Pediatric Diabetes*, *7*(4), 223–228. https://doi.org/10.1111/j.1399-5448.2006.00187.x

Puchalska, P., & Crawford, P. A. (2017). Multi-dimensional Roles of Ketone Bodies in Fuel Metabolism, Signaling, and Therapeutics. *Cell Metabolism*, *25*(2), 262–284. https://doi.org/10.1016/j.cmet.2016.12.022

Ruan, H.-B., & Crawford, P. A. (2018). Ketone bodies as epigenetic modifiers. *Current Opinion in Clinical Nutrition & Metabolic Care*, *21*(4), 260–266. https://doi.org/10.1097/MCO.0000000000000475

Sarbassov, D. D., Guertin, D. A., Ali, S. M., & Sabatini, D. M. (2005). Phosphorylation and Regulation of Akt/PKB by the Rictor-mTOR Complex. *Science*, *307*(5712), 1098–1101. https://doi.org/10.1126/science.1106148

Schafer, K. A. (1998). The Cell Cycle: A Review. *Veterinary Pathology*, *35*(6), 461–478. https://doi.org/10.1177/030098589803500601

Singh, N., Baby, D., Rajguru, J., Patil, P., Thakkannavar, S., & Pujari, V. (2019). Inflammation and cancer. *Annals of African Medicine*, *18*(3), 121. https://doi.org/10.4103/aam.aam_56_18

Srinivasan, S., Guha, M., Kashina, A., & Avadhani, N. G. (2017). Mitochondrial dysfunction and mitochondrial dynamics-The cancer connection. *Biochimica et Biophysica Acta (BBA) - Bioenergetics*, *1858*(8), 602–614. https://doi.org/10.1016/j.bbabio.2017.01.004

Sung, H., Ferlay, J., Siegel, R. L., Laversanne, M., Soerjomataram, I., Jemal, A., & Bray, F. (2021). Global Cancer Statistics 2020: GLOBOCAN Estimates of Incidence and Mortality Worldwide for 36 Cancers in 185 Countries. *CA: A Cancer Journal for Clinicians*, *71*(3), 209–249. https://doi.org/10.3322/caac.21660

Talib, W. H., Mahmod, A. I., Kamal, A., Rashid, H. M., Alashqar, A. M. D., Khater, S., Jamal, D., & Waly, M. (2021). Ketogenic Diet in Cancer Prevention and Therapy: Molecular Targets and Therapeutic Opportunities. *Current Issues in Molecular Biology*, *43*(2), 558–589. https://doi.org/10.3390/cimb43020042

Tan-Shalaby, J. (2017). Ketogenic Diets and Cancer: Emerging Evidence. *Federal Practitioner : For the Health Care Professionals of the VA, DoD, and PHS*, *34*(Suppl 1), 37S-42S.

Vettore, L., Westbrook, R. L., & Tennant, D. A. (2020). New aspects of amino acid metabolism in cancer. *British Journal of Cancer*, *122*(2), 150–156. https://doi.org/10.1038/s41416-019-0620-5

Weber, D. D., Aminazdeh-Gohari, S., & Kofler, B. (2018). Ketogenic diet in cancer therapy. *Aging*, *10*(2), 164–165. https://doi.org/10.18632/aging.101382

Weber, D. D., Aminzadeh-Gohari, S., Tulipan, J., Catalano, L., Feichtinger, R. G., & Kofler, B. (2020). Ketogenic diet in the treatment of cancer – Where do we stand? *Molecular Metabolism*, *33*, 102–121. https://doi.org/10.1016/j.molmet.2019.06.026

Wheless, J. W. (2008). History of the ketogenic diet. *Epilepsia*, *49*(s8), 3–5. https://doi.org/10.1111/j.1528-1167.2008.01821.x

Wright, C., & Simone, N. L. (2016). Obesity and tumor growth. *Current Opinion in Clinical Nutrition & Metabolic Care*, *19*(4), 294–299. https://doi.org/10.1097/MCO.0000000000000286

Zahra, A., Fath, M. A., Opat, E., Mapuskar, K. A., Bhatia, S. K., Ma, D. C., III, S. N. R., Snyders, T. P., Chenard, C. A., Eichenberger-Gilmore, J. M., Bodeker, K. L., Ahmann, L., Smith, B. J., Vollstedt, S. A., Brown, H. A., Hejleh, T. A., Clamon, G. H., Berg, D. J., Szweda, L. I., … Allen, B. G. (2017). Consuming a Ketogenic Diet while Receiving Radiation and Chemotherapy for Locally Advanced Lung Cancer and Pancreatic Cancer: The University of Iowa Experience of Two Phase 1 Clinical Trials. *Radiation Research*, *187*(6), 743–754. https://doi.org/10.1667/RR14668.1

Zhu, H., Bi, D., Zhang, Y., Kong, C., Du, J., Wu, X., Wei, Q., & Qin, H. (2022). Ketogenic diet for human diseases: the underlying mechanisms and potential for clinical implementations. *Signal Transduction and Targeted Therapy*, *7*(1), 11. https://doi.org/10.1038/s41392-021-00831-w

Chapter 6

The Ketogenic Diet and Neuroglia

Eric Uribe[1]
Carmen Rubio[1]
Vanessa Mena[1]
Noel Gallardo[1]
Diana Flores[1]
David Vázquez[1]
and Moisés Rubio-Osornio[2]

[1]Departamento de Neurofisiología, Instituto Nacional de Neurología y Neurocirugía Manuel Velasco Suárez, Mexico City, Mexico
[2]Departamento de Neuroquímica, Instituto Nacional de Neurología y Neurocirugía Manuel Velasco Suárez, Mexico City, Mexico

Abstract

Since their discovery, neuroglia cells have been believed to serve merely as support tissue for nerve cells, holding a secondary role in neurophysiology. However, as technological advances enabled more comprehensive studies, their essential role in the metabolism of the nervous microenvironment became clear. Like neurons, glia require glucose to survive and generate sufficient energy for their diverse functions. Yet, the brain can adeptly adjust to conditions of low glucose concentrations in the body, such as those seen in ketosis induced by the ketogenic diet. Astrocytes, oligodendrocytes, and other glial cells are crucial in the utilization of ketone bodies as energy substrates during ketone oxidation processes, ensuring the nervous system's metabolism adapts without compromising its homeostatic function.

In: The Ketogenic Diet Reexamined
Editors: Leticia Granados-Rojas and Carmen Rubio
ISBN: 979-8-89113-543-7
© 2024 Nova Science Publishers, Inc.

Keywords: neuroglia, ketogenic diet, metabolic oxidation, ketosis, ketone bodies

Acronyms

AcAc	Acetoacetate
AMPA	α-amino-3-hydroxy-5-methyl-4-isoxazolepropionic acid
ATP	Adenosine triphosphate
BHB	β-hydroxybutyrate
cAMP	Cyclic adenosine monophosphate
CNS	Central nervous system
CPT-I	Carnitine palmitoyltransferase I
EAAT2	Excitatory amino acid transporter 2
ENS	Enteric nervous system
G6P	Glucose-6-phosphate
GABA	Gamma-aminobutyric acid
GLS1	Glutaminase 1
GLUT	Glucose transporter
HDL	High density lipoprotein
HMG-CoA	β-Hydroxy β-methylglutaryl-CoA
IGF	Insulin like growth-factor
KB	Ketone bodies
KCC2	Potassium chloride cotransporter 2
KD	Ketogenic diet
LDH5	Lactate dehydrogenase 5
MCTs	Monocarboxylic acid transporters
NAD	Nicotinamide adenine dinucleotide
NADPH	Nicotinamide adenine dinucleotide phosphate hydrogen
NF-kB	Nuclear factor kappa B
NG-2	Neural/glial antigen 2
NH3	Ammonia
NMDA	N-methyl-D-aspartate
OPCs	Oligodendrocyte precursors
SAT	System A transport
SN-1	System N transport-1
TCA	Tricarboxylic acid
vGLUT	Vesicular glutamate transporter

Introduction

In 1856, Rudolf Virchow described glia as brain connective tissue. Earlier, in 1838, Robert Remak had identified what we now know as Schwann cells and nerve fibers. (Zhang et al., 2013)

The conformation of neuroglia is complex. Glial cells are part of the central and peripheral nervous system. It is important to note that they are non-neuronal cells; this means that they cannot create electrical driving forces. They play an essential role also in maintaining neuronal support, homeostasis regulation by controlling neurotransmitter fluxes, eliminating foreign agents by phagocytosis, and eliminating or repairing damaged neurons (Puchowicz et al., 2008)

In other words, they have a structural function and participate at a physiological level for correct neuronal functioning.

The ketogenic diet (KD) has been mentioned since Hippocrates times, as it was recognized as an epilepsy treatment. Subsequently, during the following years, various researchers continued to study this diet. In 1921, Dr. H. Rawle Geyelin was the first to demonstrate the favorable results in cognition that occurred with fasting in epileptic patients. KD, which consists of a high fat intake and a carbohydrate restriction, induces a state of ketosis in the human body. When glucose is limited, the metabolic machinery will be stimulated to compensate and adapt through alternate biochemical pathways. In order to keep the metabolic rates and energy fluxes in the organs starting from non-glucidic substrates with fatty acid oxidation to produce ketone bodies (KBs). In neuroscience, ketosis oxidative metabolism in the brain has been documented to cause changes in mitochondrial function and influence neurotransmitter release. KBs as energy substrates increase hyperpolarization at the membrane potential and affect the synthesis of gamma-aminobutyric acid (GABA) while simultaneously decreasing the release of glutamate and norepinephrine (Rudy et al., 2020; Sampaio, 2016).

The molecular and biochemical role of neuroglia in oxidative metabolism induced by the KD and its interaction within the neural microenvironment will be described throughout the chapter. Emphasis will be placed on the direct effect of KD on the different types of glial cells populations, including the biological effects and clinical benefits of KD.

Neuroglia and the Ketogenic Diet

The study and understanding of the nervous system functioning have been a subject of human interest since ancient times. Brain understanding approached a cellular level in the second half of the 19th century when the principles of neuronal theories were born. Back in 1858, Rudolf Virchow, father of modern pathology, described a series of structures arranged between the neuronal tissue, joining or linking nerve cells to each other, which is why he defined it as neuroglia (from the Greek glia, glue) (Fan & Agid, 2018). At that time, glia was nothing more than a kind of connective tissue that maintained the neuronal structure, with a secondary role compared to the well-known neurons. It was Santiago Ramón y Cajal, Nobel Prize winner, who in 1891 projected neuroglia as a tissue that goes beyond its role of support, postulating that these group of cells were differentiated from neurons, thus proposing a more relevant position within the nervous system (Li et al., 2020)

Since Ramón y Cajal postulates, glia have been studied with more detail, and what has been found is surprising since their role in neurophysiology is increasingly relevant.

At almost the same time, scientists described glia fundamentals; scientists worldwide were already working on studying ketosis processes and their role within the nervous system. The first scientific work, already exploring the ketogenesis process's influence on the brain, was done in 1910 in France. It described how the seizures ended during absolute fasting. Shortly after, in 1921, Russel Wilder, a Mayo Clinic physician, used the KD to treat epileptical disorders and studied prolonged ketosis in diabetic patients. After World War II episodes, scientists like Dr. Livingston and Dr. Hopkins analyzed a clinical sample of 1,000 patients who presented seizures and reported their control using this diet (Wheless, 2008).

To understand the biochemical and molecular effects of KD on neuroglia, it is essential that we briefly remember their functions within the nervous system. Thus, glia differentiate from neuronal cells due to their lack of axons, and because they are silent cells, i.e., they do not have action potentials or synaptic potentials. Furthermore, the glia outnumber the neurons by a ratio of approximately 3:1, occupying almost 50% of the total brain volume. The aforementioned characteristics are of utmost importance because these will cause the glia to fill in the spaces around neurons, and this intimate relationship between them will cause the glia to be actively involved in all neuronal signaling processes. We can classify neuroglia (Table 1) into histologically distinct and, hence, functionally different populations (Adel K. Afifi & Ronald A. Bergman, 2020; López-Gómez et al., 2021)

As we can see, neuroglia has a strategic anatomical arrangement that allows them to collaborate with neurons to perform homeostatic maintenance of the nervous microenvironment, participating in various functions such as local nutrition, modulation of synaptic activity, or cell defence and repair (Lukacova et al., 2021).

As discussed later, ketosis have an active role in the nervous system, so its metabolic and biochemical action affect the glia. KD, which will biochemically force the body to opt for a pro-ketonic state, consists of eating high fats, moderate proteins, and restricted carbohydrates (Dhamija et al., 2013). Under normal physiological circumstances, our cells consume carbohydrates, primarily glucose, as an oxidative substrate to obtain energy by generating adenosine triphosphate (ATP) molecules through glycolysis (Prince et al., 2013). When we reduce the intake of glucose, the primary metabolic fuel source, under certain nutritional conditions like starvation, fasting, development, or a ketogenic diet (KD) feeding, metabolic effectors such as insulin decrease their secretion. This leads the body into a catabolic state, activating metabolic processes like ketogenesis, fatty acid oxidation, and gluconeogenesis. As a result, alternative energy substrates like KBs step in to fulfill the body's basal metabolic rate (Roehl et al., 2019).

We can now understand that ketosis is the cellular biochemical method in which carbohydrate intake depletion provokes the degradation of fat in ketone bodies by hepatic fatty acid oxidation in a process known as ketogenesis, as can be seen in Figure 1 (Fukao et al., 2004).

Nowadays, KD is among the most popular nutritional experts worldwide due to the advantages that have been demonstrated mainly for clinical improvement of diverse pathological situations, including neurological diseases. Evidence has shown different biological benefits when the body is subjected to ketosis through this diet, as shown in Table 2. It has an active role in reducing the inflammatory cascade and metabolic stress by activating the sequencing of single-cell RNA in adipocytes and T cells, thus is a practical strategy not only for weight loss but for decreasing metabolic syndrome effects and systemic inflammation. Other tested advantages of this diet are positive changes in the human gastrointestinal system by improving its microbiome state (Dowis & Banga, 2021; Rivière et al., 2016)

It can also change the structure of the epigenome by modifying the chromatin structure, increasing gene expression in DNA repair and DNA methylation, and preventing chronic and metabolic diseases through these genetic mechanisms (Miller et al., 2018). It contributes to growth inhibition in cancer cells by modifying the ability of glucose usage in this cell (Dąbek et al., 2020) and can also improve lipid profile levels by modifying atherogenic factors (Shai et al., 2008).

Table 1. Main functions of different types of glia

Type of glia cell	Localization	Function
Fibrous astrocyte	CNS: White matter	Metabolite's transfer Healing damaged tissue by a neurotrophic function
Protoplasmic astrocyte	CNS: Gray matter	Metabolic intermediators for nerve cells
Radial glial cell	CNS: Throughout the brain during development	Allows neuronal precursor migration to the different regions of the brain by its projections
Müller cell	CNS: Retina	Regulates glutamate influx and modulates the activity of retinal photoreceptor cells. Composition control of extracellular fluid Regenerative and neuronal plasticity capabilities
Bergmann glia	CNS: Cerebellar cortex	Glutamate uptake and extracellular K+ homeostasis Calcium transient passage in presence of glutamate Membrane potential regulator of cerebellar Purkinje cells
Ependymal cell	CNS: Ventricular lining	Formation of cerebrospinal fluid. Neurosecretion functions in the subcommissural organ
Oligodendrocyte	CNS: Mainly in white matter but also found in gray matter	Myelin sheath synthesis in CNS. Neuronal growth inhibition Brain pH and iron regulation
Schwann cell	PNS: Peripheral axons	Protection and axonal metabolic support Contribute to nerve conduction processes and regeneration mechanisms of injured axons.
Microglia	CNS: Throughout the brain	Phagocytic capacity Promotes neural cell survival, proliferation, and differentiation in adult CNS development.
NG-2 positive glia	CNS: Pons, somatosensory cortex, thalamus cortex, cerebellum and hippocampus	Precursors of oligodendrocytes, astrocytes and even neurons under certain conditions Only glial cells capable of receiving synaptic contacts. Key role in the glial scar formation
Enteric glial cell	ENS: Intestinal wall	Intestinal barrier support Gastrointestinal motility Active role in visceral sensation May act as a reactive proinflammatory phenotype
Satellite cell	PNS: Sensory and autonomic ganglia	Microenvironment homeostasis by regulating the molecular diffusion across the cell membrane. Neurotransmission regulation by transporters

NG-2: Neural/Glial antigen 2; CNS: Central nervous system; PNS: Peripheral nervous system; ENS: Enteric nervous system.

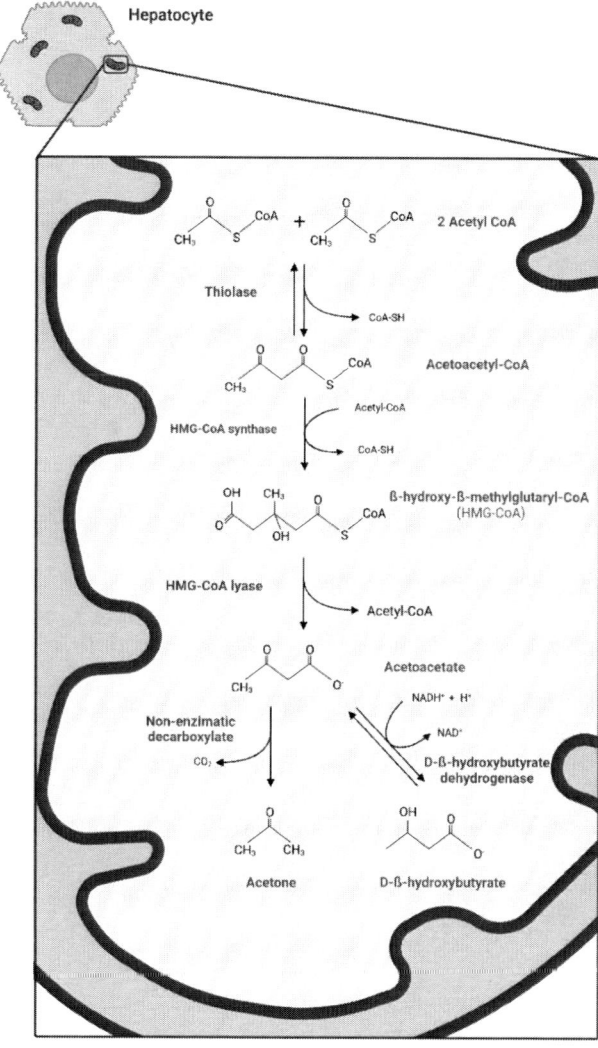

Figure 1. Ketogenesis: In the presence of a high rate of fatty acid oxidation in the liver, mitochondria use acetyl-CoA from ß-oxidation to convert it into ketone bodies; acetone, acetoacetate, and D-ß-hydroxybutyrate, which are subsequently transported by blood to peripheral tissues to be used as alternative fuel. Initially, a thiolase inversion occurs where 2 moles of acetyl-CoA are converted to acetoacetyl-CoA, then HMG-CoA synthase combines a third molecule of acetyl-CoA with acetoacetyl-CoA to produce HMG-CoA. Finally, HMG-CoA under the action of HMG-CoA lyase produces acetoacetate and acetyl-CoA. Acetoacetate undergoes a NADH-dependent reduction to give rise to D-ß-hydroxybutyrate or, after spontaneous decarboxylation, produces acetone, which is not biologically metabolized and can be eliminated in respiration. HMG-CoA synthase: β-hydroxy-β-methylglutaryl-CoA synthase.

Table 2. Biological and clinical benefits of ketogenic diet

Biological effect	Clinical effect
Reduces inflammation and metabolic stress	↓Metabolic syndrome effects
	↓Systemic inflammation
Improves neurochemical signal of GABA in neurons	↓Seizures and ↑prognosis of refractory epilepsy
Increases *Bacteroidetes* and *Bifidobacteria* species	Improves gastrointestinal function by helping its microbiome´s balance
Influences aerobic metabolism on mitochondrial respiration and decrease oxidative stress	Prevention of neurodegenerative and other chronic diseases
Decreasing in the ketolytic enzymes in cancer cells and in the IGF	↓Cancer risk
	Inhibits cancer proliferation
Modification in the atherogenic lipid profile: ↓ triglycerides, ↓ total cholesterol, ↑HDL levels	↓Cardiovascular risk
	Better dyslipidemia and blood glucose control

GABA: gamma-aminobutyric acid; IGF: Insulin like growth-factor; HDL: High density lipoprotein.

In the neuroscience field, the effects of induced ketosis have been studied in many neurological diseases, epilepsy being one of the most researched areas. Several have concluded that it may be able to improve the prognosis of refractory epilepsy by improving the neurochemical signal of GABA in neurons and influencing aerobic metabolism in mitochondrial respiration; as mentioned above, changes in the epigenome can also help prevent neurodegenerative diseases (Gzielo et al., 2019; Gzielo et al., 2020). Yet there are still questions: How does the ketosis process affect glial physiology? Is there a direct interrelationship between KD and neuroglia?

Ketosis and Brain Metabolism

As mentioned in the introduction, when the metabolic energy of the body is forced into a ketosis state, the liver will be responsible for acetyl CoA formation through fatty acid beta-oxidation. As ketosis is perpetuated and oxaloacetate depleted by the high demand for glucose production, acetyl CoA will accumulate and stimulate the formation of KB, which will abandon the liver circulation to be used in the brain. Once in the brain, KBs must be reactivated into acetoacetyl CoA to enter the tricarboxylic acid (TCA) cycle and produce energy or synthesize amino acids (Fedotova et al., 2021; Melø et al., 2006). Two of the three KBs produced in ketogenesis interest us for their role in neuron-glia oxidation: acetoacetate (AcAc) and β-hydroxybutyrate (BHB).

Speaking of AcAc, Zhang et al. (2013) used it along with glucose because both are biochemical substrates for energy production through the Krebs cycle, to demonstrate, by stable isotope mass spectrometry analysis, the brain's ability to switch from glucose towards KB cortical oxidation with chronic ketosis, proving that cerebral metabolic rate for glucose decreases as ketosis increases when rats were induced in a 3 week KD (cortical brain utilized twice as much AcAc in chronic induced ketosis). In fact, approximately 70% of neuronal CO_2 production comes from AcAc degradation, while in astrocytes, a not insignificant percentage of 40% comes from the same process (Pan et al., 2002). Another key AcAc mechanism studied in the ketotic state is the decrease in neuronal excitability by reducing presynaptic glutamate release at the synaptic cleft, as it modulates glutamate vesicles release (Lebon et al., 2002). A neuroprotective effect will be triggered because, in the context of oxidative stress in the brain, ketosis stabilizes glucose metabolism by partitioning brain glucose away from oxidative metabolism towards KB oxidation, controlling the alteration of glucose metabolism that occurs in situations such as epilepsy or ischemic reperfusion injury (Puchowicz et al., 2008).

BHB is another well-known KB that the CNS uses as an alternative energy pathway known as ketolysis. It has been reported that in the brain of rats its consumption is relatively small, being only 3% of total basal metabolism. However, in obese patients who fasted for three weeks, it was observed that this KB provides a major fraction of brain oxidative metabolism, reported at approximately 50% of the energy produced (Gjedde & Crone, 1975). Although this ketone has been shown to be oxidized to a greater extent by neuronal metabolism in the context of hyperketonemia, astrocytes cannot be left out of the equation, as their consumption for the oxidation of BHB alone is 20% (Afridi et al., 2020). The oxidation model of BHB between the neuron-astrocyte complex is very interesting because the tripartite synapse is involved in the energy flows of this ketone. We know that astrocytes primarily manage the concentration of glutamate in the extracellular fluid to prevent its over accumulation and subsequent neuronal injury. It is precisely in this relationship between both cells that the oxidative flow of BHB occurs (Figure 2), first entering the neuron and then going to the astrocytic pools after the metabolism to glutamate by ketolysis (Boison & Steinhäuser, 2018). There is no doubt that it is necessary to consider the quantitative astrocytic contributions of KBs oxidation as fractional enrichers of glutamate and glutamine (Lukacova et al., 2021; Pan et al., 2002).

Regarding GABA in the context of chronic ketosis, there are two mechanisms that stimulate its function in the central nervous system (CNS). In the first instance, its synthesis is substantially increased in states of hyperketonemia, neurons convert KBs to acetyl CoA, increasing the flux toward the reaction with citrate synthase to the TCA cycle, provoking the oxaloacetate to be consumed and therefore less available for the reaction with aspartate aminotransferase. Physiologically, this will mean that less glutamate is converted to aspartate, exposing glutamate to reactions with glutamine synthetase and glutamate decarboxylase (Lizarbe et al., 2019). In the second mechanism, the expression increase observed in potassium chloride cotransporter 2 (KCC2) in the dentate gyrus and cortex of rats increases the inhibitory strength of GABA (Granados-Rojas et al., 2020; Murakami & Tognini, 2022).

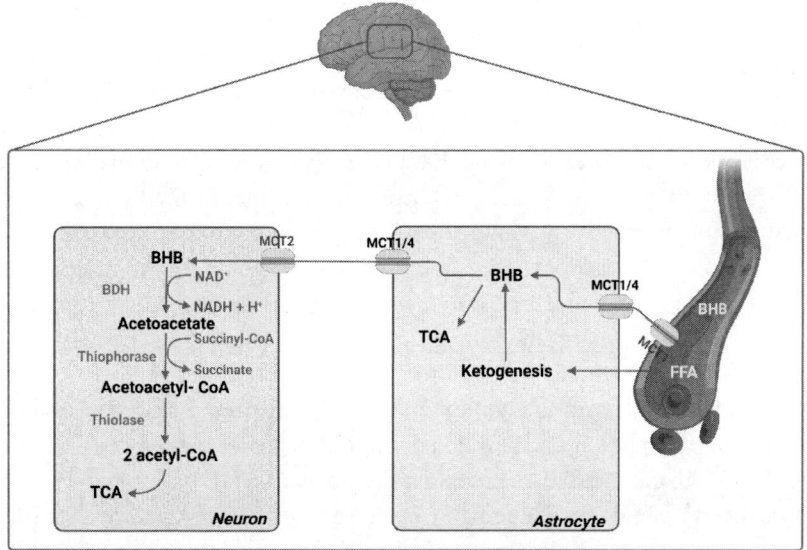

Figure 2. Neuron-glia oxidative flow of BHB: In the brain, astrocytes have the capacity to develop ketogenesis, starting from the fatty acids coming from blood to produce ketone bodies. Also, D-BHB is directly uptake by astrocytes through blood MCT1/4. Once the ketone bodies have been upheld and produced, they go to neurons crossing MCT2 where BHB is oxidized to acetoacetate by BHB dehydrogenase, producing NADH. Then acetoacetate is activated by thiophorase to form acetoacetyl-CoA. Reconversion involves the enzymatic transfer of a CoA moiety from succinyl-CoA to acetoacetate to give acetoacetyl-CoA. With the addition of a CoA, acetoacetyl-CoA is cleaved into 2 moles of acetyl-CoA by thiolase and oxidized in the citric acid cycle. BHB: β-hydroxybutyrate.

We have discussed so far how KBs are produced to reach the nervous territory so they can interact with brain cells for their metabolism through oxidation, where they can function correctly in glucose-deprived situations as a form of adaptation to the nervous microenvironment. However, we have yet to define the role of the different types of glia in ketones' oxidative metabolism. There are several studies that have effectively demonstrated the involvement of KB production in improving neuroglial cell function, especially within the central and peripheral nervous system.

Ketosis and the Different Types of Neuroglia

Astrocytes

Astrocytes are the most abundant glial cells in the brain, so their role in the function of the CNSis essential. Among their most notable functions, there is the regulation of neurotransmitters, the maintenance of water homeostasis, the supply of neurons with substrates for oxidative phosphorylation, and the regulation of blood supply to meet neuronal energy demand (Bordone et al., 2019). These glial cells are characterized by terminal feet surrounding brain arteries and capillaries, as well as extensive processes originating from the soma, the latter of which envelop the synapses, forming a functional unit called a tripartite synapse. This neurometabolic coupling is one of the fundamental parts in understanding neuroenergetics since it takes place within neurons and the astrocyte, sharing their metabolic pathways so they may cover their basal energetic rates.

Physiologically, glucose is taken up from cerebral microvessels by GLUT1 channels on the astrocyte's terminal foot covering them. Almost instantaneously, glucose is phosphorylated to glucose-6-phosphate (G6P) by the enzyme hexokinase I, routing G6P into three possible pathways: into the glycolysis pathway to produce pyruvate, metabolized to glucose-1-phosphate for glycogen synthesis, or used in the pentose phosphate pathway. The latter route generates NADPH, an essential molecule for maintaining antioxidant-reduced glutathione and as a precursor for nucleotide synthesis. Without ketogenesis and ketolysis, astrocytes can use lactate as an alternative substrate to glucose within the hypothesis of lactate shuttle hypothesis (Figure 3) (Bordone et al., 2019).

Astrocytes are the main site of fatty acid oxidation in the CNS. Thus, the metabolic effect of KD in the brain is practically done within this glial population. This cellular adaptation allows the use of KBs as oxidizable fuel for neurons in caloric restriction environments. As a result of the nutritional ketosis state, there is an effect on the astrocytic glutamate-glutamine cycle, on glutamate synthase activity, and on the vesicular glutamate transporter function (Morris, Maes, et al., 2020).

As we previously mentioned, KBs and lactate participate as the main alternative energy stores, and both have been shown to be able to efficiently cross the blood-brain barrier through monocarboxylate transporters (MCTs) expressed in endothelial cells and astroglia. It has been noted that after a prolonged fast of more than 4 weeks, KB levels increase significantly and can enhance and increase total brain energy reserves by more than 50% (Jensen et al., 2020).

In ketotic animals, astrocytes have a more active metabolism of acetate, also reflected in increased pyruvate recycling in glutamate. The conversion of acetate to acetyl CoA is more active in astrocytes, and their acetate uptake and intracellular processing is also increased too (Melø et al., 2006). A genetic effect has also been observed in this type of cell glia; it was shown that when serum glucose levels decreased, the expression of insulin pathway genes was altered; after exposure to prolonged fasting, astrocytes showed a decrease in the expression, unlike neurons that showed a significant increase (Koppel et al., 2021).

Astrocytes interact with neurons by synaptic cleft activity, enhancing neurotransmitter production to maintain adequate neuronal excitability; in this scenario, an increased lactate supply has been evidenced under conditions of high synaptic activity. Similarly, an increase in cyclic adenosine monophosphate (cAMP) concentrations has been found, which under normal conditions will activate glycolysis, glycogen mobilization, and, in the same way, under prolonged fasting conditions, will activate ketogenesis in astrocytes (Thevenet et al., 2016). Through cAMP activation, astrocytes would induce the production of KBs that would notably prevent irreversible detrimental damage to nonesterified fatty acids that would have a cerebral neuroprotective effect; in collaboration with lactate, ketones would participate in the decrease of neuronal death (Guzmán & Blázquez, 2001).

Surprisingly, in astrocyte cultures, it has been found that they can metabolize KBs and produce them from leucine and fatty acids. This evidence concludes that the ketogenic machinery of astrocytes can be compared to that of hepatocytes for three reasons: The ketogenic capacity of both is similar as they show a preference for fatty acids over glucose as the main fuel, producing large amounts of KBs; the ketogenesis function of both is to mitochondrially regulated by carnitine palmitoyltransferase I (CPT-I), which catalyzes the rate-setting step of the biochemical process and that both cell groups share the same properties of their CPT-I, thus being an isoenzyme which is inhibited mainly by malonyl-CoA levels in both tissues (Guzmán & Blázquez, 2004).

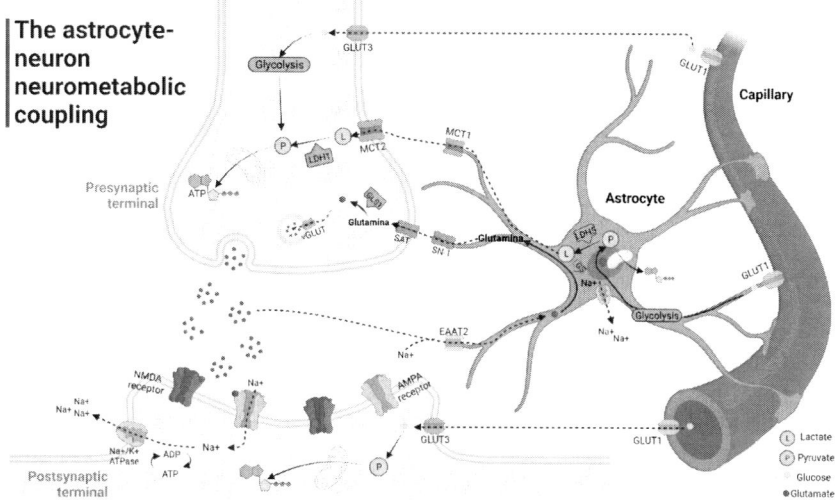

Figure 3. The astrocyte-neuron neurometabolic coupling: Representation of the energy expenditure in the glutamate-glutamine cycle and the astrocyte-neuron lactate shuttle hypothesis. Vesicular glutamatergic release activates two receptors in postsynaptic neurons, which are AMPA and NMDA. This depolarizes the membrane by opening channels, triggering the influx of Na^+ ions, using ATP when they are pumped out through the Na+/K+ ATPase pump. Glutamate left in the synaptic cleft is taken up in astrocytes by EAAT2 to be metabolized via glutamine synthase. Glutamine produced in the glial cell is released through SN-1 and neurons will absorb it via SAT to replenish glutamate pools through GLS1 and vesicular reuptake through vGLUT. Most of the energy required by these presynaptic and postsynaptic processes comes from glycolysis, although neurons and glia can use alternative energy substrates. Glucose uptake will be held by astrocytes from blood capillaries through GLUT1 to convert to lactate by LDH5 to be released and taken up by neurons through MCT. Neurons convert lactate to pyruvate by LDH1, which enters the TCA cycle and is metabolized by oxidative phosphorylation in mitochondria. AMPA: α-amino-3-hydroxy-5-methyl-4-isoxazolepropionic acid. NMDA: N-methyl-D-aspartate. EAAT2: excitatory amino acid transporter 2. SN-1: system N transport-1. SAT: system A transport. GLS1: glutaminase 1. vGLUT: vesicular glutamate transporter. GLUT: glucose transporter 1. LDH5: lactate dehydrogenase 5. MCT: monocarboxylic acid transporters. LDH1: lactate dehydrogenase 1. TCA: Tricarboxylic acid.

Microglia and NG-2 Positive Glia

Microglia, as immune cells of the CNS, perform their functions through a surveillance system and rapid response, being able to monitor and regulate changes in neuronal activity and contributing to the structure of neuronal networks and their connectivity. This is possible thanks to coordinated processes that make transitory contact with synaptic and extra-synaptic areas and with the presence of receptors for neuromodulators, such as neurotransmitters, cytokines, and chemokines (Morris, Puri, et al., 2020).

For the correct functioning of microglia, a high energy demand is required where the main energy substrates are glucose, fatty acids, and glutamine. Glucose enters the microglia via GLUT1, GLUT3, GLUT4 and GLUT5 to later be used in glycolysis and complete aerobic breakdown or can be used in the formation and secretion of lactate. It should be noted that fatty acids can serve as an alternative energy source for microglia. After lipase uptake, acyl-CoA synthetase catalyzes the formation of fatty acyl-CoA in the mitochondria, where it is b-oxidized to acetyl-CoA and finally enters the TCA cycle and later the electron transport chain to generate ATP. On the other hand, microglia express SLC1A5 and SLC38A1 transporters that allow microglia to uptake glutamine. Once inside the mitochondria, glutamine is turned into glutamate and ammonia (NH_3) by glutaminase. Finally, so that glutamate can enter the TCA cycle, it is metabolized by glutamate dehydrogenase 1 to α-ketoglutarate (Ghosh et al., 2018).

Otherwise, during periods of prolonged fasting or starvation, microglia have the capacity to absorb KBs (BHB and AcAc) through MCT (MCT1 and MCT2) to be used as an alternative source of energy. In these periods, the expression of MCTs in the blood-brain barrier and KBs in the blood is increased.

KD and fasting have reported anti-inflammatory effects, including suppression of microglial activation (Morris, Maes, et al., 2020). It has been shown that BHB is able to inhibit histone deacetylation and activate specific receptors for microglia, such as GRP109A (HCA2) (Ghosh et al., 2018). The above decreases nuclear factor kappa B (NF-kB) signaling and pro-inflammatory cytokine production. Therefore, it would be implicated in improving this immunological function as well as their maturation, serving as a neuroprotective factor in microglia´s different phenotypes (Chen et al., 2019; Rahman et al., 2014; Zeng et al., 2021).

Other experimental studies have found that ketosis could inhibit microglia activation and promote oligodendrocyte precursors (OPCs) or neural/glial antigen 2 (NG-2) positive glia to migrate and proliferate in damaged tissue such as in chronic demyelination processes, triggering a protective effect against insufficient remyelination management, as seen in diseases like multiple sclerosis where there is a protection of myelin from toxic and pro-inflammatory effects and stimulating OPCs mature into oligodendrocytes (Li et al., 2020; N. Zhang et al., 2020).

Schwann Cells and Oligodendrocytes

Oligodendrocytes are cells located within the CNS that can act as a means of producing the myelin sheath that surrounds axons in this system. Myelin will act as an electrical insulator against noxious stimuli, increasing the resistance of the membrane and adept at decreasing its capacitance. Due to this, there will be an effective conduction velocity modification by generating a notable increase and, therefore, an effective benefit in generating an adequate translation of the electrical impulses. Similarly, oligodendrocytes have been found to participate in the supply of lactate to axons. Several studies have found that the myelination process is a relevant cycle that will depend on abundant energy reserves due to the increased demand for proteins and lipids necessary concentration for the generation of myelin (Bordone et al., 2019).

Myelinating cells such as Schwann cells and oligodendrocytes require high levels of fatty acids to generate the lipids that make up myelin. Studies have shown that approximately 20% of the total energy expenditure of the brain is occupied by β oxidation. Such is the need for these myelinating cells, as well as astrocytes, to have an energy profile in which fatty acid oxidation and aerobic glycolysis are regulated by each other (Poitelon et al., 2020). Mitochondrial dysfunction in Schwann cells has been reported to cause axonal degeneration accompanied by demyelination (Viader et al., 2013).

KD has been proposed as part of the management of demyelinating diseases in peripheral nerves, as in the case of diabetic neuropathy, where both myelinated and unmyelinated peripheral nerve fibers would be affected (Stumpf et al., 2019). It has been evidenced that liver KB production improved some of the mitochondrial anomalies in Schwann cells and the axonal functional capacity, including nonmyelinated axons; clinically speaking, after being induced in an 8-week KD, said effect improved sensory alterations such as allodynia. It was also found to be a protective myelin mechanism by regulating metabolic imbalance and predisposition to increase in the formation of reactive oxygen species, avoiding all axonal injury (Bouçanova & Chrast, 2020; Har-Even et al., 2021).

Other Glial Cells

Müller cells are the main type of glial cells in the retina, and their functions are diverse, but fundamentally they are responsible for the metabolic and homeostatic support of neurons in the retina. Among these mechanisms is the regulation of extracellular fluid composition by transcellular control of concentrations of ions such as calcium or potassium, as well as bicarbonate and water (Reichenbach & Bringmann, 2013). Although, their ability to oxidize KB is not described, it is theoretically possible. This type of glia is known to have a mechanism very similar to that of astrocytes in the removal of most of the glutamate from the extracellular site produced in the retina continuously by photoreceptor cells in the dark phase for the transmission of visual signals. For the Müller cell to generate biochemical products such as glutamine, alanine, or α-ketoglutarate from the capture of GABA, glutamate, and ammonium, glucose is required as an energy substrate (Bringmann et al., 2009). In the context of chronic ketosis, where glucose is no longer sufficient to meet energy needs, Müller cells can make use of KBs within ketogenesis to adapt metabolically, as astrocytes do.

Another minimally studied glial cell group is the ependymal cells, also known as tanycytes, which have specialized functions depending on the region in the CNS where they are located. The tanycytes that have been more widely studied are those belonging to the hypothalamus. Rather than acting as regulators of the extracellular liquid of the parenchyma, such as astrocytes, they are chemosensory cells that sense the composition of cerebrospinal fluid in the third ventricle to regulate the energy balance from this neuroanatomical region (Bolborea & Langlet, 2021). Hypothalamic ependymal cells are mainly glucosensitive, where in the presence of glucose, an activation response of the P2Y1 receptor will elicit calcium signals that propagate across the tanycyte membrane, and ATP release. Their gating function is due to the fact that tanycytes have functional tight junction proteins, causing them not only to uptake glucose but also to have selective lipid uptake along with the blood-brain barrier cells. Consequently, hypothalamic tanycytes will set individual thresholds for glucose utilization versus specific fatty acid oxidation (Bolborea & Dale, 2013). They also have an adaptive response to high-fat diets such as KD as, together with astrocytes, it enhances β-oxidation and ketogenesis pathways, ultimately producing KBs. Although the capacity for oxidationbeta oxidation in tanycytes is still unknown, it is clear that this glial group also has a ketogenic function for cellular adaptation, where in symbiosis with astrocytes they supply energy to the locoregional microenvironment (Hofmann et al., 2017; Takeda et al., 2021).

Conclusion

Undoubtedly, the discovery of glia has revolutionized the understanding of the nervous system functioning and its relationship with metabolism. We know that glia participates in many processes involving the balance of neuronal activity and other biological pathways.

The KD induces a chronic state of ketosis from which the brain can adapt, using KBs to obtain energy. AcAc and BHB will pass through the blood-brain barrier to act as metabolic effectors in neurons and glial cells; as a result, a potentiation of glial cells will be stimulated, improving their functions and allowing them to trigger neuroprotection and repair processes against lesions of the central and peripheral nervous system. Furthermore, KD has demonstrated a variety of positive effects in other pathologies such as neurodegenerative and chronic diseases, decreased cardiovascular and cancer risk, and reduced inflammatory cascade and metabolic stress.

Oxidative metabolism of KB in neuroglia will lead to up-regulation and reuse of neurotransmitters neurotransmitter secretion, such as glutamate and GABA, as well as stimulation of cell maturation in the case of NG-2 positive glia and inhibition of immune response-induced microglia injury, among others discussed throughout this chapter. We must inquire about the role of neuroglia in metabolic pathways such as ketosis and their relationship with already known pathophysiological processes. Only then can we formulate new alternative therapeutic targets using glia as our ally.

Disclaimer

None.

Acknowledgments

We thank the Armstrong Foundation for the undergraduate scholarship to David Vázquez.

References

Adel K. Afifi, & Ronald A. Bergman. (2020). *Neurohistología [Neurohistology]." Neuroanatomía Funcional: Texto y Atlas* . McGrawHill.

Afridi, R., Kim, J.-H., Rahman, M. H., & Suk, K. (2020). Metabolic Regulation of Glial Phenotypes: Implications in Neuron–Glia Interactions and Neurological Disorders. *Frontiers in Cellular Neuroscience*, *14*. https://doi.org/10.3389/fncel.2020.00020

Boison, D., & Steinhäuser, C. (2018). Epilepsy and astrocyte energy metabolism. *Glia*, *66*(6), 1235–1243. https://doi.org/10.1002/glia.23247

Bolborea, M., & Dale, N. (2013). Hypothalamic tanycytes: potential roles in the control of feeding and energy balance. *Trends in Neurosciences*, *36*(2), 91–100. https://doi.org/10.1016/j.tins.2012.12.008

Bolborea, M., & Langlet, F. (2021). What is the physiological role of hypothalamic tanycytes in metabolism? *American Journal of Physiology-Regulatory, Integrative and Comparative Physiology*, *320*(6), R994–R1003. https://doi.org/10.1152/ajpregu.00296.2020

Bordone, M. P., Salman, M. M., Titus, H. E., Amini, E., Andersen, J. V., Chakraborti, B., Diuba, A. V., Dubouskaya, T. G., Ehrke, E., Espindola de Freitas, A., Braga de Freitas, G., Gonçalves, R. A., Gupta, D., Gupta, R., Ha, S. R., Hemming, I. A., Jaggar, M., Jakobsen, E., Kumari, P., ... Seidenbecher, C. I. (2019). The energetic brain – A review from students to students. *Journal of Neurochemistry*, *151*(2), 139–165. https://doi.org/10.1111/jnc.14829

Bouçanova, F., & Chrast, R. (2020). Metabolic Interaction Between Schwann Cells and Axons Under Physiological and Disease Conditions. *Frontiers in Cellular Neuroscience*, *14*. https://doi.org/10.3389/fncel.2020.00148

Bringmann, A., Pannicke, T., Biedermann, B., Francke, M., Iandiev, I., Grosche, J., Wiedemann, P., Albrecht, J., & Reichenbach, A. (2009). Role of retinal glial cells in neurotransmitter uptake and metabolism. *Neurochemistry International*, *54*(3–4), 143–160. https://doi.org/10.1016/j.neuint.2008.10.014

Chen, F., He, X., Luan, G., & Li, T. (2019). Role of DNA Methylation and Adenosine in Ketogenic Diet for Pharmacoresistant Epilepsy: Focus on Epileptogenesis and Associated Comorbidities. *Frontiers in Neurology*, *10*. https://doi.org/10.3389/fneur.2019.00119

Dąbek, A., Wojtala, M., Pirola, L., & Balcerczyk, A. (2020). Modulation of Cellular Biochemistry, Epigenetics and Metabolomics by Ketone Bodies. Implications of the

Ketogenic Diet in the Physiology of the Organism and Pathological States. *Nutrients*, *12*(3), 788. https://doi.org/10.3390/nu12030788

Dhamija, R., Eckert, S., & Wirrell, E. (2013). Ketogenic Diet. *Canadian Journal of Neurological Sciences / Journal Canadien Des Sciences Neurologiques*, *40*(2), 158–167. https://doi.org/10.1017/S0317167100013676

Dowis, K., & Banga, S. (2021). The Potential Health Benefits of the Ketogenic Diet: A Narrative Review. *Nutrients*, *13*(5), 1654. https://doi.org/10.3390/nu13051654

Fan, X., & Agid, Y. (2018). At the Origin of the History of Glia. *Neuroscience*, *385*, 255–271. https://doi.org/10.1016/j.neuroscience.2018.05.050

Fedotova, A. A., Tiaglik, A. B., & Semyanov, A. V. (2021). Effect of Diet as a Factor of Exposome on Brain Function. *Journal of Evolutionary Biochemistry and Physiology*, *57*(3), 577–604. https://doi.org/10.1134/S0022093021030108

Fukao, T., Lopaschuk, G. D., & Mitchell, G. A. (2004). Pathways and control of ketone body metabolism: on the fringe of lipid biochemistry. *Prostaglandins, Leukotrienes and Essential Fatty Acids*, *70*(3), 243–251. https://doi.org/10.1016/j.plefa.2003.11.001

Ghosh, S., Castillo, E., Frias, E. S., & Swanson, R. A. (2018). Bioenergetic regulation of microglia. *Glia*, *66*(6), 1200–1212. https://doi.org/10.1002/glia.23271

Gjedde, A., & Crone, C. (1975). Induction processes in blood-brain transfer of ketone bodies during starvation. *American Journal of Physiology-Legacy Content*, *229*(5), 1165–1169. https://doi.org/10.1152/ajplegacy.1975.229.5.1165

Granados-Rojas, L., Jerónimo-Cruz, K., Juárez-Zepeda, T. E., Tapia-Rodríguez, M., Tovar, A. R., Rodríguez-Jurado, R., Carmona-Aparicio, L., Cárdenas-Rodríguez, N., Coballase-Urrutia, E., Ruíz-García, M., & Durán, P. (2020). Ketogenic Diet Provided During Three Months Increases KCC2 Expression but Not NKCC1 in the Rat Dentate Gyrus. *Frontiers in Neuroscience*, *14*. https://doi.org/10.3389/fnins.2020.00673

Guzmán, M., & Blázquez, C. (2001). Is there an astrocyte–neuron ketone body shuttle? *Trends in Endocrinology & Metabolism*, *12*(4), 169–173. https://doi.org/10.1016/S1043-2760(00)00370-2

Guzmán, M., & Blázquez, C. (2004). Ketone body synthesis in the brain: possible neuroprotective effects. *Prostaglandins, Leukotrienes and Essential Fatty Acids*, *70*(3), 287–292. https://doi.org/10.1016/j.plefa.2003.05.001

Gzielo, K., Janeczko, K., Węglarz, W., Jasiński, K., Kłodowski, K., & Setkowicz, Z. (2020). MRI spectroscopic and tractography studies indicate consequences of long-term ketogenic diet. *Brain Structure and Function*, *225*(7), 2077–2089. https://doi.org/10.1007/s00429-020-02111-9

Gzielo, K., Soltys, Z., Rajfur, Z., & Setkowicz, Z. K. (2019). The Impact of the Ketogenic Diet on Glial Cells Morphology. A Quantitative Morphological Analysis. *Neuroscience*, *413*, 239–251. https://doi.org/10.1016/j.neuroscience.2019.06.009

Har-Even, M., Rubovitch, V., Ratliff, W. A., Richmond-Hacham, B., Citron, B. A., & Pick, C. G. (2021). Ketogenic Diet as a potential treatment for traumatic brain injury in mice. *Scientific Reports*, *11*(1), 23559. https://doi.org/10.1038/s41598-021-02849-0

Hofmann, K., Lamberz, C., Piotrowitz, K., Offermann, N., But, D., Scheller, A., Al-Amoudi, A., & Kuerschner, L. (2017). Tanycytes and a differential fatty acid metabolism in the hypothalamus. *Glia*, *65*(2), 231–249. https://doi.org/10.1002/glia.23088

Jensen, N. J., Wodschow, H. Z., Nilsson, M., & Rungby, J. (2020). Effects of Ketone Bodies on Brain Metabolism and Function in Neurodegenerative Diseases. *International Journal of Molecular Sciences*, *21*(22), 8767. https://doi.org/10.3390/ijms21228767

Koppel, S. J., Pei, D., Wilkins, H. M., Weidling, I. W., Wang, X., Menta, B. W., Perez-Ortiz, J., Kalani, A., Manley, S., Novikova, L., Koestler, D. C., & Swerdlow, R. H. (2021). A ketogenic diet differentially affects neuron and astrocyte transcription. *Journal of Neurochemistry*, *157*(6), 1930–1945. https://doi.org/10.1111/jnc.15313

Lebon, V., Petersen, K. F., Cline, G. W., Shen, J., Mason, G. F., Dufour, S., Behar, K. L., Shulman, G. I., & Rothman, D. L. (2002). Astroglial Contribution to Brain Energy Metabolism in Humans Revealed by ^{13}C Nuclear Magnetic Resonance Spectroscopy: Elucidation of the Dominant Pathway for Neurotransmitter Glutamate Repletion and Measurement of Astrocytic Oxidative Metabolism. *The Journal of Neuroscience*, *22*(5), 1523–1531. https://doi.org/10.1523/JNEUROSCI.22-05-01523.2002

Li, R., Zhang, P., Zhang, M., & Yao, Z. (2020). The roles of neuron-NG2 glia synapses in promoting oligodendrocyte development and remyelination. *Cell and Tissue Research*, *381*(1), 43–53. https://doi.org/10.1007/s00441-020-03195-9

Lizarbe, B., Cherix, A., Duarte, J. M. N., Cardinaux, J.-R., & Gruetter, R. (2019). High-fat diet consumption alters energy metabolism in the mouse hypothalamus. *International Journal of Obesity*, *43*(6), 1295–1304. https://doi.org/10.1038/s41366-018-0224-9

López-Gómez, L., Szymaszkiewicz, A., Zielińska, M., & Abalo, R. (2021). Nutraceuticals and Enteric Glial Cells. *Molecules*, *26*(12), 3762. https://doi.org/10.3390/molecules26123762

Lukacova, N., Kisucka, A., Kiss Bimbova, K., Bacova, M., Ileninova, M., Kuruc, T., & Galik, J. (2021). Glial-Neuronal Interactions in Pathogenesis and Treatment of Spinal Cord Injury. *International Journal of Molecular Sciences*, *22*(24), 13577. https://doi.org/10.3390/ijms222413577

Melø, T. M., Nehlig, A., & Sonnewald, U. (2006). Neuronal–glial interactions in rats fed a ketogenic diet. *Neurochemistry International*, *48*(6–7), 498–507. https://doi.org/10.1016/j.neuint.2005.12.037

Miller, V. J., Villamena, F. A., & Volek, J. S. (2018). Nutritional Ketosis and Mitohormesis: Potential Implications for Mitochondrial Function and Human Health. *Journal of Nutrition and Metabolism*, *2018*, 1–27. https://doi.org/10.1155/2018/5157645

Morris, G., Maes, M., Berk, M., Carvalho, A. F., & Puri, B. K. (2020). Nutritional ketosis as an intervention to relieve astrogliosis: Possible therapeutic applications in the treatment of neurodegenerative and neuroprogressive disorders. *European Psychiatry*, *63*(1), e8. https://doi.org/10.1192/j.eurpsy.2019.13

Morris, G., Puri, B. K., Maes, M., Olive, L., Berk, M., & Carvalho, A. F. (2020). The role of microglia in neuroprogressive disorders: mechanisms and possible neurotherapeutic effects of induced ketosis. *Progress in Neuro-Psychopharmacology and Biological Psychiatry*, 99, 109858. https://doi.org/10.1016/j.pnpbp.2020.109858

Murakami, M., & Tognini, P. (2022). Molecular Mechanisms Underlying the Bioactive Properties of a Ketogenic Diet. *Nutrients*, *14*(4), 782. https://doi.org/10.3390/nu14040782

Pan, J. W., de Graaf, R. A., Petersen, K. F., Shulman, G. I., Hetherington, H. P., & Rothman, D. L. (2002). [2,4-^{13}C$_2$]-β-Hydroxybutyrate Metabolism in Human Brain. *Journal of Cerebral Blood Flow & Metabolism*, *22*(7), 890–898. https://doi.org/10.1097/00004647-200207000-00014

Poitelon, Y., Kopec, A. M., & Belin, S. (2020). Myelin Fat Facts: An Overview of Lipids and Fatty Acid Metabolism. *Cells*, *9*(4), 812. https://doi.org/10.3390/cells9040812

Prince, A., Zhang, Y., Croniger, C., & Puchowicz, M. (2013). *Oxidative Metabolism: Glucose Versus Ketones* (pp. 323–328). https://doi.org/10.1007/978-1-4614-7411-1_43

Puchowicz, M. A., Zechel, J. L., Valerio, J., Emancipator, D. S., Xu, K., Pundik, S., LaManna, J. C., & Lust, W. D. (2008). Neuroprotection in Diet-Induced Ketotic Rat Brain after Focal Ischemia. *Journal of Cerebral Blood Flow & Metabolism*, *28*(12), 1907–1916. https://doi.org/10.1038/jcbfm.2008.79

Rahman, M., Muhammad, S., Khan, M. A., Chen, H., Ridder, D. A., Müller-Fielitz, H., Pokorná, B., Vollbrandt, T., Stölting, I., Nadrowitz, R., Okun, J. G., Offermanns, S., & Schwaninger, M. (2014). The β-hydroxybutyrate receptor HCA2 activates a neuroprotective subset of macrophages. *Nature Communications*, *5*(1), 3944. https://doi.org/10.1038/ncomms4944

Reichenbach, A., & Bringmann, A. (2013). New functions of Müller cells. *Glia*, *61*(5), 651–678. https://doi.org/10.1002/glia.22477

Rivière, A., Selak, M., Lantin, D., Leroy, F., & De Vuyst, L. (2016). Bifidobacteria and Butyrate-Producing Colon Bacteria: Importance and Strategies for Their Stimulation in the Human Gut. *Frontiers in Microbiology*, *7*. https://doi.org/10.3389/fmicb.2016.00979

Roehl, K., Falco-Walter, J., Ouyang, B., & Balabanov, A. (2019). Modified ketogenic diets in adults with refractory epilepsy: Efficacious improvements in seizure frequency, seizure severity, and quality of life. *Epilepsy & Behavior*, *93*, 113–118. https://doi.org/10.1016/j.yebeh.2018.12.010

Rudy, L., Carmen, R., Daniel, R., Artemio, R., & Moisés, R.-O. (2020). Anticonvulsant mechanisms of the ketogenic diet and caloric restriction. *Epilepsy Research*, *168*, 106499. https://doi.org/10.1016/j.eplepsyres.2020.106499

Sampaio, L. P. de B. (2016). Ketogenic diet for epilepsy treatment. *Arquivos de Neuro-Psiquiatria*, *74*(10), 842–848. https://doi.org/10.1590/0004-282X20160116

Shai, I., Schwarzfuchs, D., Henkin, Y., Shahar, D. R., Witkow, S., Greenberg, I., Golan, R., Fraser, D., Bolotin, A., Vardi, H., Tangi-Rozental, O., Zuk-Ramot, R., Sarusi, B., Brickner, D., Schwartz, Z., Sheiner, E., Marko, R., Katorza, E., Thiery, J., … Stampfer, M. J. (2008). Weight Loss with a Low-Carbohydrate, Mediterranean, or

Low-Fat Diet. *New England Journal of Medicine*, *359*(3), 229–241. https://doi.org/10.1056/NEJMoa0708681

Stumpf, S. K., Berghoff, S. A., Trevisiol, A., Spieth, L., Düking, T., Schneider, L. V., Schlaphoff, L., Dreha-Kulaczewski, S., Bley, A., Burfeind, D., Kusch, K., Mitkovski, M., Ruhwedel, T., Guder, P., Röhse, H., Denecke, J., Gärtner, J., Möbius, W., Nave, K.-A., & Saher, G. (2019). Ketogenic diet ameliorates axonal defects and promotes myelination in Pelizaeus–Merzbacher disease. *Acta Neuropathologica*, *138*(1), 147–161. https://doi.org/10.1007/s00401-019-01985-2

Takeda, H., Yamaguchi, T., Yano, H., & Tanaka, J. (2021). Microglial metabolic disturbances and neuroinflammation in cerebral infarction. *Journal of Pharmacological Sciences*, *145*(1), 130–139. https://doi.org/10.1016/j.jphs.2020.11.007

Thevenet, J., De Marchi, U., Domingo, J. S., Christinat, N., Bultot, L., Lefebvre, G., Sakamoto, K., Descombes, P., Masoodi, M., & Wiederkehr, A. (2016). Medium-chain fatty acids inhibit mitochondrial metabolism in astrocytes promoting astrocyte-neuron lactate and ketone body shuttle systems. *The FASEB Journal*, *30*(5), 1913–1926. https://doi.org/10.1096/fj.201500182

Viader, A., Sasaki, Y., Kim, S., Strickland, A., Workman, C. S., Yang, K., Gross, R. W., & Milbrandt, J. (2013). Aberrant Schwann Cell Lipid Metabolism Linked to Mitochondrial Deficits Leads to Axon Degeneration and Neuropathy. *Neuron*, *77*(5), 886–898. https://doi.org/10.1016/j.neuron.2013.01.012

Wheless, J. W. (2008). History of the ketogenic diet. *Epilepsia*, *49*(s8), 3–5. https://doi.org/10.1111/j.1528-1167.2008.01821.x

Zeng, H., Lu, Y., Huang, M.-J., Yang, Y.-Y., Xing, H.-Y., Liu, X.-X., & Zhou, M.-W. (2021). Ketogenic diet-mediated steroid metabolism reprogramming improves the immune microenvironment and myelin growth in spinal cord injury rats according to gene and co-expression network analyses. *Aging*, *13*(9), 12973–12995. https://doi.org/10.18632/aging.202969

Zhang, N., Liu, C., Zhang, R., Jin, L., Yin, X., Zheng, X., Siebert, H.-C., Li, Y., Wang, Z., Loers, G., & Petridis, A. K. (2020). Amelioration of clinical course and demyelination in the cuprizone mouse model in relation to ketogenic diet. *Food & Function*, *11*(6), 5647–5663. https://doi.org/10.1039/C9FO02944C

Zhang, Y., Kuang, Y., LaManna, J. C., & Puchowicz, M. A. (2013). *Contribution of Brain Glucose and Ketone Bodies to Oxidative Metabolism*(pp. 365–370). https://doi.org/10.1007/978-1-4614-4989-8_51

Chapter 7

The Regional Expression of NKCC1 Cotransporter in the Dentate Gyrus of Rats Fed with a Ketogenic Diet

Karina Jerónimo-Cruz[1,2]
Tarsila Elizabeth Juárez-Zepeda[2]
Joyce Graciela Martínez-Galindo[3]
Miguel Tapia-Rodríguez[4]
America Vanoye Carlo[2]
and Leticia Granados-Rojas[2],*

[1]Laboratorio de Bioquímica y Endocrinología, Instituto Nacional de Pediatría, Mexico City, Mexico
[2]Laboratorio de Neurociencias II, Instituto Nacional de Pediatría, Mexico City, Mexico
[3]Laboratorio de Demencias, Instituto Nacional de Neurología y Neurocirugía, Manuel Velasco Suárez, Mexico City, Mexico
[4]Unidad de Microscopía, Instituto de Investigaciones Biomédicas, Universidad Nacional Autónoma de México, Mexico City, Mexico

Abstract

Ketogenic diet (KD) is a dietary regimen rich in fat, low in carbohydrates and adequate in protein. Initially, the diet was used as a non-pharmacological treatment in refractory epilepsy. However, in recent time, the diet has been shown to be effective in treating various neurological and psychiatric diseases associated with gamma aminobutyric acid (GABA) neurotransmitter dysfunction. NKCC1 is a

---

* Corresponding Author's Email: lgranados_2000@yahoo.com.mx.

In: The Ketogenic Diet Reexamined
Editors: Leticia Granados-Rojas and Carmen Rubio
ISBN: 979-8-89113-543-7
© 2024 Nova Science Publishers, Inc.

cotransporter responsible for chloride inflow into the neurons. Thus, it participates in the regulation of intracellular chloride concentration that determines the effect of neurotransmission mediated by GABA. This study aimed to compare the regional distribution pattern of NKCC1 cotransporter expression in the dorsal/ventral and right/left dentate gyrus of rats fed with KD during a period from weaning to three months post-weaning. At the beginning and the end of the treatment, the body weight and the blood levels of glucose and β-hydroxybutyrate were measured. In addition, the expression of NKCC1 was analyzed by estimating the number of NKCC1 immunoreactive (NKCC1-IR) cells by stereological methods using the optical fractionator technique. At the end of treatment, the results indicated that the blood levels of β-hydroxybutyrate were higher in KD-fed rats. However, the stereological count of NKCC1-IR cells in these rats did not show any difference in their regional distribution pattern in the dorsal/ventral and right/left dentate gyrus. These findings show that a three-month application of KD does not affect NKCC1 cation-chloride cotransporter expression in the dentate gyrus regions of the rats.

Keywords: ketogenic diet, NKCC1, dentate gyrus, stereology, optical fractionator, laterality, rat

Acronyms

ANOVA	Analysis of Variance
BrdU	Thymidine analog 5-bromodeoxyuridine
CA1	*Cornus Ammonis* 1
CA3	*Cornus Ammonis* 3
CICUAL	Institutional Committee for the Care and Use of Laboratory Animals
Cl$^-$	Chloride anion
DAB	3,3'-diaminobenzidine
DG	Dentate gyrus
DR	Dorsal region
DR-LH	Dorsal region of the left hemisphere
DR-RH	Dorsal region of the right hemisphere
GABA	Gamma-aminobutyric acid
GL	Granule layer
HL	Hilus
K$^+$	Potassium cation
KA	Kainic acid

KCC2	Cation-chloride cotransporter K^+-Cl^- 2
KD	Ketogenic diet
LH	Left hemisphere
ML	Molecular layer
Na^+	Sodium cation
ND	Normal diet
NKCC1	Cation-chloride cotransporter Na^+-K^+-$2Cl^-$ 1
NKCC1-IR	NKCC1 immunoreactivity
NKCC2	Cation-chloride cotransporter Na^+-K^+-$2Cl^-$ 2
P	Postnatal
PB	Phosphate buffer
PFA	Paraformaldehyde in phosphate buffer
RH	Right hemisphere
SE	Standard error
SPSS	Statistical package for social sciences
SUB	Subiculum
USA	United States of America
VR	Ventral region
VR-LH	Ventral region of the left hemisphere
VR-RH	Ventral region of the right hemisphere

Introduction

Ketogenic diet (KD) is a high-fat, low-carbohydrate, and adequate protein dietary regimen widely recognized as a biochemical model of fasting (Fedorovich et al., 2018).

Fasting and other dietary regimens have been used to treat epilepsy since 500 BC (Wheless, 2008). In 400 BC, Hippocrates proposed fasting (complete abstinence from food and drink) as an effective method for the treatment of epilepsy. In the bible, similar descriptions of fasting as an efficacious cure for epilepsy are also found (Gulati, 2018). Lately, in the 1920s, KD was introduced to mimic the metabolism of fasting as a treatment for epilepsy (Wheless, 2008). The term KD was first mentioned by Wilder, at Mayo Clinic, in 1921, who applied KD on trial for the treatment of epilepsy. Also, in the same year, Geyelin et al. reported an 87% success (seizure-free) in a cohort of 30 patients after a 20-day fasting (Wheless, 2004).

As the pharmacological investigation for broad-spectrum highly effective antiepileptic drugs evolved, with the discovery of phenytoin in 1938 and sodium valproate in 1970, the popularity of KD weaned off, becoming restricted only to difficult cases such as Lennox-Gastaut syndrome (Wheless, 2008).

KD replaces carbohydrates with fats, inducing the production of ketone bodies (acetoacetate, acetone and β-hydroxybutyrate) from fatty acids; thus, replacing glucose, the main energy substrate for neurons, with ketone bodies. These ketone bodies are carried to the brain through the bloodstream, where acetoacetate and β-hydroxybutyrate are metabolized in the mitochondria to yield energy. β-hydroxybutyrate is the predominant ketone body. Classic KD composes of a 4:1 macronutrient ratio, that is, 4 grams of fat per gram of protein and carbohydrates (McDonald & Cervenka, 2018).

Recent evidence shows that KD is effective in the treatment of several diseases, such as obesity (Paoli, 2014; Choi et al., 2020), mitochondrial dysfunctions (Kang et al., 2007; Qu et al., 2021), cancer (Seyfried et al., 2012; Plotti et al., 2020) and aging (Balietti et al., 2010). It is also effective in neurological (Stafstrom & Rho, 2012) and psychiatric diseases (Bostock et al., 2017) that are associated with gamma aminobutyric acid regulated-neurotransmission dysfunction.

The cation-chloride cotransporters, Na^+-K^+-$2Cl^-$ 1 (NKCC1) and K^+-Cl^- 2 (KCC2), transport chloride into and out of neurons respectively. Hence, they regulate intracellular chloride concentration, which determines the effect of gamma aminobutyric acid (GABA) (Kahle et al., 2008).

The gene family SLC12 of electroneutral cation-chloride cotransporters contains NKCC1 glycoprotein (Kaila et al., 2014; Koumangoye et al., 2021). The *SLC12A2* gene located on the long arm of the chromosome 5 at 5q23.3 encodes NKCC1 cotransporter, which has two isoforms: A and B (Meor & Zhang, 2020; Koumangoye et al., 2021). NKCC1 and NKCC2 use sodium and potassium as cations to couple to chloride transport. In the plasma membrane of epithelial and non-epithelial cells, the homeostasis of K^+, Na^+, and Cl^- is maintained by NKCC1 and NKCC2 (Meor & Zhang, 2020; Xie et al., 2020). NKCCs are reciprocally regulated by kinases and phosphatases (Koumangoye et al., 2021); therefore, they are activated by phosphorylation and inactivated by dephosphorylation (Delpire & Gagnon, 2018; Koumangoye et al., 2021).

GABA is the main inhibitory neurotransmitter of the cerebral cortex; however, it can act as an exciter due to the high concentration of Cl^- ions and low concentration of K^+, regulated by the cotransporters NKCC1 and KCC2. This, hypoexcitability or hyperexcitability of neurons has been related to diverse pathologies, such as neuropathic pain, edema after an ischemic brain injury, and temporal lobe epilepsy (Kahle et al., 2008; Kahle et al., 2010), among others.

The mechanism of action of KD is unspecified. However, it has been suggested that its action is due to the changes in the expression of the NKCC1 and/or KCC2 cotransporter (Granados-Rojas et al., 2020). This study aimed to compare the regional distribution pattern of the NKCC1 cotransporter expression in dorsal/ventral and right/left dentate gyrus of rats fed with a KD for three months starting from the weaning period.

Methods

Animals and Diets

All experimental procedures developed in the research reported in this chapter followed the guidelines of the Official Mexican Norm for the use and care of laboratory animals (NOM-062-ZOO-1999) and belonged to protocol 085-2010, approved by the Research Board of the National Institute of Pediatrics and by the Institutional Committee for the Care and Use of Laboratory Animals (CICUAL).

Sixteen male Sprague-Dawley rats bred and kept under constant controlled conditions of temperature (22-24°C), relative humidity (40%) and light:dark cycle (12:12 h) were used. Filter air (5 mm particles) was exchanged 18 times in 1 h. The rats were divided in two groups (control and experimental groups) each with eight rats. The control group, here called ND group, was fed with a normal diet (2018S sterilized, Envigo Teklad, United States of America (USA) and the experimental group, here named KD group, was fed with ketogenic diet (TD 96355, Envigo Teklad, USA). Prior to the dietary treatments, the animals of KD group were subjected to one-day fasting. Both groups have access to water *ad libitum* during this period and the rest of the experiment. The diets were provided during three months beginning on postnatal (P) day 21 for ND group and P22 for KD group, until P112. Table 1 shows the composition of the diets based on weight and energy content of each one.

In blood samples obtained via tail vein, the blood levels of glucose and β-hydroxybutyrate were measured at the beginning (P21 or P22) and the end (P112) of the treatments, the body weight was also measured. The glucose and β-hydroxybutyrate were determined with a glucometer and test strips (Abbott Laboratories).

Table 1. Nutritional composition of diets

Nutrients (% by weight)	Normal diet 2018S Envigo Teklad	Ketogenic diet TD.96355 Envigo Teklad
Protein	18.60	15.30
Fat	6.20	67.40
Carbohydrate	44.20	0.50
Energy (kcal/g)	3.10	6.70

Tissue Processing and Immunocytochemical Staining

Tissue processing and immunocytochemical staining were performed as previously reported by Granados-Rojas et al. (2020). Briefly, at the end of treatment the animals were anesthetized with sodium pentobarbital (50 mg/kg, intraperitoneally) and euthanized via transcardial perfusion with 0.9% NaCl solution followed by 4% paraformaldehyde in phosphate buffer (PB), 0.1 M, pH 7.4 (PFA). After 24 h of fixation in PFA, brains were cryoprotected with a sucrose gradient. Brain coronal serial sections were cut at 50 μm on a cryostat (Leica, Germany). To select the sections to be evaluated from each serial slides, a systematic random procedure was used, and this consists of selecting one of every eight sections, giving a total of 11-16 sections of whole rat dentate gyrus.

An immunohistochemistry protocol was carried out to evaluate the expression of the cation-chloride cotransporter NKCC1 using a secondary biotinylated antibody according to Brandt et al. (2010) in parallel free-floating at room temperature, and simultaneously using the same conditions. Briefly, sections were initially washed three times with PBS with each of the washes lasting 10 min, between the change of each solution and at the end. The sections were subsequently processed with 1% hydrogen peroxide in PBS for 10 minutes. Later, the tissues were incubated with 20X ImmunoDNA retriever buffer (Bio SB, USA) for 60 min and followed by an overnight incubation with primary rabbit polyclonal antibodies anti-NKCC1 (1:500; Merck-Millipore, Germany, AB3560P), which recognizes total protein. Subsequently, sections were washed and incubated with a secondary biotinylated goat anti-rabbit biotinylated IgG antibody (1:500; Vector Laboratories, USA, BA-1000) for two h and incubated with avidin peroxidase complex (ABC kit; Vectastain; Vector Laboratories, USA, Pk-4000) for one h. Finally, the staining was revealed with 3,3'-diaminobenzidine (DAB; Vector Laboratories, USA, SK-4100) for two and a half min. The tissue was mounted onto poly-L-lysine-coated slides. The primary antibody NKCC1 and the secondary biotinylated antibody were omitted as negative controls to assess nonspecific binding in additional sections (Granados-Rojas et al., 2020).

Stereology

To count the number of NKCC1 immunoreactive (NKCC1-IR) cells in different regions of the layers of the dentate gyrus of both DN and KD-fed rats, an optical fractionator, a stereological systematic random procedure (West et al. al., 1991) was used. Stereo Investigator 9 software on a semi-automated stereological system (MBF Bioscience, Vermont, USA) was used. The characteristics of the counting frame were as follows: size, 70 × 45 µm; dissector height 13 µm and the definition of the guard zones at 1.5 µm from the upper and lower edges of the counting frame. The grid size was set to 300 × 300 µm, except for the granular layer, which was set to 250 × 250 µm. Cell counting was performed with a 60X objective (Granados-Rojas et al., 2020). The error coefficient (Gundersen, m = 1) was <0.1.

NKCC1-IR cells number were counted separately in molecular, granule and hilus layers of the dentate gyrus. Measurements were made in the dentate gyrus of the left (LH) and right (RH) hemispheres to determine if there were differential changes in the number of NKCC1-IR cells by laterality. The determination of differential changes per region was assessed by counting the number of NKCC1-IR cells in the dorsal (DR), (-1.72 to -4.08 mm posterior to Bregma) and ventral region (VR), (-4.20 to -6.8 mm posterior to Bregma) (Paxinos & Watson, 2007), obtaining the following zones of analysis:

1. Dorsal region of the left hemisphere (DR-LH).
2. Dorsal region of the right hemisphere (DR-RH).
3. Ventral region of the left hemisphere (VR-LH).
4. Ventral region of the right hemisphere (VR-RH).
5. Total left hemisphere (Total LH: DR-LH + VR-LH).
6. Total right hemisphere (Total RH: DR-RH + VR-RH).
7. Total dorsal region (Total DR: DR-LH + DR-RH).
8. Total ventral region (Total VR: VR-LH + VR-RH).

Statistical Analysis

Data from body weight, glucose and β-hydroxybutyrate were subjected to separate two-way mixed Analysis of Variance (ANOVA) that included the between-subject factor: Group (ND *vs* KD) and the within-subject factor: Time (initial *vs* final measure).

The NKCC1-IR cells count in the hilus, molecular and granule layers of the dentate gyrus were subjected to separate mixed three-way ANOVAs, that include the between-subject factor Group (ND *vs* KD), and the within factors: Hemisphere (right *vs* left) and Region (dorsal *vs* ventral). Only interactions that include the Group factor are reported.

For all analyses, Mauchly's sphericity test was performed. Furthermore, as the test indicated no sphericity ($p < 0.05$) for all cases, the Greenhouse-Geisser correction method was used. In addition, significant interactions were analyzed with Bonferroni's *post-hoc* test. For these cases, the original degrees of freedom and the corrected probability levels are reported as well as the partial eta square. For all analyses, the significance level was maintained at $p < 0.05$. All analyses were performed with the statistical package for social sciences (SPSS), version 20.

Results

Body Weight

Assessment of body weight was performed at the beginning and end of the study. In this study, the KD-fed rats tolerated their diet well for three months, and the body weights of ND and KD group rats continuously increased along the treatment. The mixed ANOVA results indicated that the interaction Group × Time was not significant $F(1, 14) = 0.540$, $p = 0.474$, which means there were no diet effects on body weight.

Glucose

The glucose mean ± standard error (SE) for ND and KD groups in each measurement are depicted in Figure 1A. The mixed ANOVA results for this variable indicated that the interaction Group × Time was not significant $F(1, 14) = 0.069$, $p = 0.797$, which means that no diet effects on glucose were observed at the beginning and end of the study.

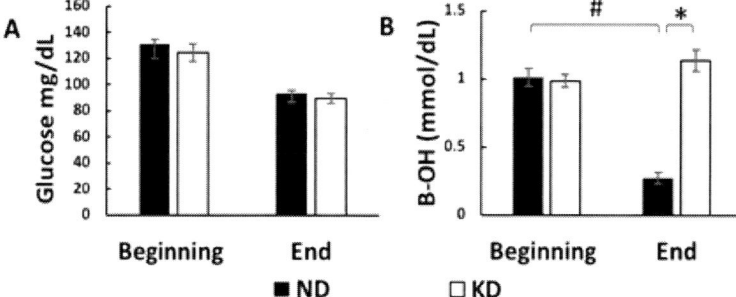

Figure 1. Quantification of glucose (**A**) and β-hydroxybutyrate (**B**). The graphs show the mean and standard error in each parameter of rats fed with normal diet (ND) or ketogenic diet (KD), both at the beginning and at the end of treatment. There were no significant differences between the two groups at the beginning and at the end in glucose levels. However, there was a significant decrease in β-hydroxybutyrate at the end of the experiment with respect to the beginning for the ND group (# $p < 0.001$) and a significant increase in the β-hydroxybutyrate KD group compared with the ND group at the end of the experiment (* $p < 0.05$). n = 8 in each group.

β-Hydroxybutyrate

Quantification of blood β-hydroxybutyrate was performed at the beginning and end of the study. The β-hydroxybutyrate mean ± SE for ND and KD groups in each measurement are depicted in Figure 1B. The mixed ANOVA showed that the interaction Group × Time was significant $F(1, 14) = 41.039$, $p < 0.001$, $\eta^2 = 0.746$. The Bonferroni's test indicated that there was a significant β-hydroxybutyrate concentration decrease at the end of the experiment with respect to the beginning for the ND group (# $p < 0.001$), but for the KD group, there were no significant changes ($p = 0.145$). As expected, the Bonferroni's test indicated that at the beginning of the study, there were no significant differences ($p = 0.752$) between ND and KD groups, but at the end of the experiment, the KD group presented a greater β-hydroxybutyrate concentration than the ND group (* $p < 0.001$).

NKCC1 Immunoreactivity

The NKCC1-IR cells mean ± SE quantified in the different zones of analysis of each layer of the dentate gyrus for ND and KD groups are shown in Figure 2.

In the molecular layer of dentate gyrus, the mixed ANOVA indicated that the Group × Hemisphere × Region interaction was not significant $F(1, 14) = 3.399$, $p = 0.088$. Similarly, the other interactions that included the Group factor were not significant: Region × Group $F(1, 14) = 0.000$, $p = 0.992$; Hemisphere × Group $F(1, 14) = 2.670$, $p = 0.126$. Also, no main effect by Group was observed $F(1, 14) = 0.628$, $p = 0.442$.

In the granule layer of the dentate gyrus, the mixed ANOVA showed no significant Group × Hemisphere × Region interaction $F(1, 14) = 0.054$, $p = 0.819$. Likewise, the other interactions that included the Group factor were not significant: Region × Group $F(1, 14) = 0.001$, $p = 0.972$; Hemisphere × Group $F(1, 14) = 0.030$, $p = 0.866$. No main effect by Group was observed $F(1, 14) = 0.033$, $p = 0.860$.

Lastly, in the dentate gyrus hilus, the mixed ANOVA results showed that the Group × Hemisphere × Region interaction was also non-significant for this layer $F(1, 14) = 0.011$, $p = 0.918$. In the same way, the other interactions that included the Group factor were not significant: Region × Group $F(1, 14) = 0.044$, $p = 0.837$; Hemisphere × Group $F(1, 14) = 0.945$, $p = 0.349$. No main effect by Group was observed $F(1, 14) = 1.298$, $p = 0.275$.

Discussion

To our knowledge, this is the first study that analyzes the regional distribution pattern of NKCC1 cotransporter expression through comparisons between dorsal/ventral region and right/left hemisphere of the molecular, granule and hilus layers of dentate gyrus of rats fed with KD.

The regional results presented in this study confirm our previously reported research, which indicate that rats fed with KD in the short (Gómez-Lira et al., 2011) and long term (Granados-Rojas et al., 2020) do not show differences in the quantification of the total number of NKCC1-IR cells in the whole layers of dentate gyrus.

Likewise, other studies in rats have not reported any effect of KD on the cotransporter NKCC1. For instance, Wang et al. (2016) did not report differences in NKCC1 protein levels in the cerebral cortex after a four-week KD administration. In other studies where electrophysiological parameters of animals treated with KD were evaluated, such as in Stafstrom et al. (1999), no alterations in synaptic transmission and neuronal excitability in the *Cornus Ammonis* 1 (CA1) area of the hippocampus were reported.

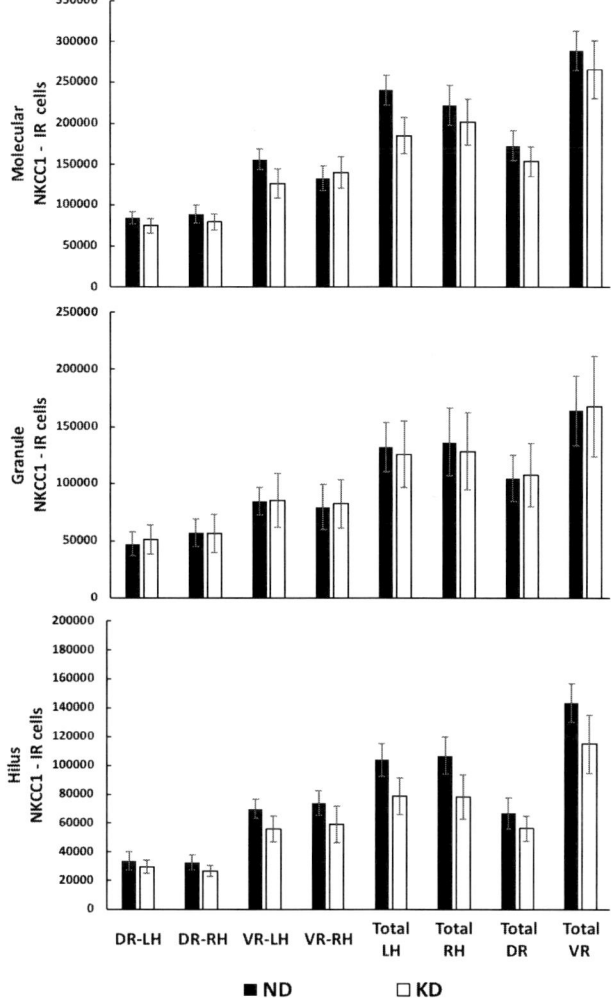

Figure 2. Quantification of NKCC1 immunoreactive (NKCC1-IR) cells number estimated by stereology of all the zones of analysis in the molecular, granule layer and hilus of the dentate gyrus of rats fed with normal diet (ND) or ketogenic diet (KD). Bar graphs show mean and standard error. There were no significant differences in the number of NKCC1-IR cells between ND and KD in any of the zones of analysis in each layer of the dentate gyrus. DR-LH: Dorsal region of the left hemisphere. DR-RH: Dorsal region of the right hemisphere. VR-LH: Ventral region of the left hemisphere. VR-RH: Ventral region of the right hemisphere. Total LH: Total left hemisphere (DR-LH + VR-LH). Total RH: Total right hemisphere (DR-RH + VR-RH). Total DR: Total dorsal region (DR-LH + DR-RH). Total VR: Total ventral region (VR-LH + VR-RH).

Nevertheless, in a previous study of our laboratory, a differential effect on the expression of cation-chloride KCC2 was observed in rats fed with a ketogenic diet for three months; specifically, an increase in the granule layer and hilus of the dentate gyrus (Granados-Rojas et al. 2020). In line with the above, is the report of Wang et al. (2016) of an increase in the expression of KCC2 cotransporter in the cerebral cortex of rats fed with KD for a month.

The cotransporters NKCC1 and KCC2 (main chloride importer and exporter respectively) are the main regulators of intracellular chloride concentration that determines the effect of GABA-mediated neurotransmission. It is probably, at least in part, that the increase in KCC2 but not NKCC1 cotransporter is associated with the beneficial effect of KD in diseases, such as epilepsy, schizophrenia, and autism spectrum disorder, etc., where GABAergic system and dentate gyrus are damaged.

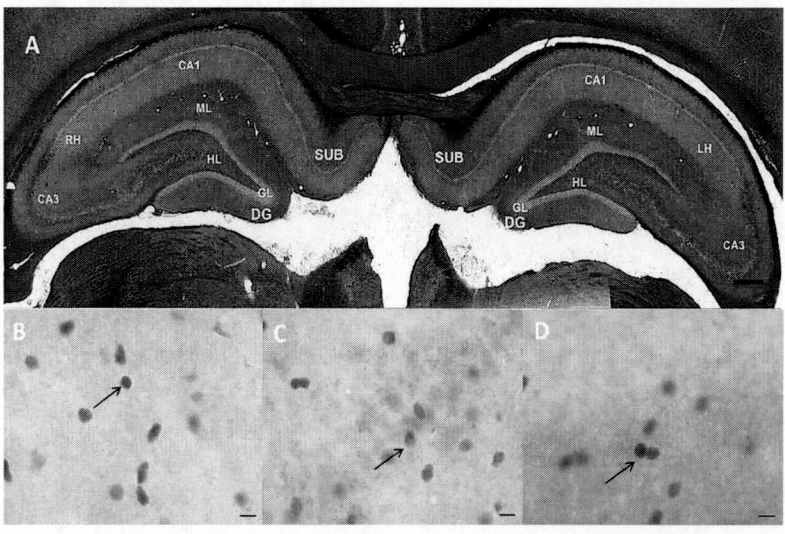

Figure 3. **A,** panoramic image of the hippocampal formation marked with NKCC1 of a rat fed with normal diet. Right hemisphere (RH) and left hemisphere (LH). The dentate gyrus (DG) lamination: molecular (ML), granule (GL) and hilus (HL) layer and the different areas of the hippocampus: *Cornus Ammonis* 1 (CA1), *Cornus Ammonis* 3 (CA3) and subiculum (SUB) are observed. NKCC1-IR cells (arrows) were found distributed through all dentate gyrus. **B,** magnification of molecular layer, **C** granule layer, and **D** hilus. Scale bar: 500 μm (A), 15 μm (B–D).

Kwon et al., (2008) investigated the effects of KD on neurogenesis after kainic acid (KA)-induced seizures in mice through quantitative analysis of thymidine analog 5-bromodeoxyuridine (BrdU) labeling. They showed an increase in the proliferation rate of neuronal progenitor cells after KA-induced seizures in the KD-fed mice but not in the seizure-free KD-fed group. Thus, the authors established the possibility that the effects of KD could reach an optimal state in hyperexcitability states. Hence, the results of the present study do not rule out the possibility of NKCC1 as a target of KD in hyperexcitable states, such as epilepsy.

The measurement of blood levels of β-hydroxybutyrate in blood samples, obtained via the tail vein at the end of the experiment, showed that KD group presented a higher concentration than the ND group. This result indicated that the KD used in the present study produces a state of ketosis after its consumption for three months, and that it is an effective diet.

The dentate gyrus is part of the hippocampal formation, a limbic system structure responsible for learning and memory processes. In rodents, the DG is divided into the dorsal and ventral region. Although the two regions are made up of the same cellular elements, they present connectivity and functional differences. The importance of analyzing the dentate gyrus lies in the fact that it is considered a "gate," since it controls and transmits information from the entorhinal cortex to the hippocampus. Additionally, the dorsal dentate gyrus has been implicated in the development of psychiatric disorders, such as depression and anxiety (Moser & Moser, 1998; Strange et al., 2014; Sun et al., 2023).

Thus, in this chapter, the effect of KD on the regional distribution pattern of NKCC1 cotransporter expression in different zones of the dorsal/ventral regions of the dentate gyrus was analyzed. Nevertheless, no significant differences were observed in the NKCC1-IR cells number in any of the zones analyzed.

Finally, the hippocampus is one of the brain areas that shows laterality: right/left with morphological asymmetries (Hami et al., 2014). However, the analysis of NKCC1-IR cells number per hemisphere in the different zones did not reveal any difference.

Conclusion

KD provided during three months does not affect the regional distribution pattern of NKCC1 cotransporter expression, since the expression in the molecular, granule and hilus layers of dentate gyrus of the dorsal/ventral region and right/left hemisphere did not how any differences. However, we suggest that more studies in this respect be conducted in other brain regions under these conditions to reach a conclusive generalization on this effect of KD.

Acknowledgments

This work was supported by Program E022 of the National Institute of Pediatrics (Ministry of Health), Protocol 85/2010 to LG-R. 86784 CONACYT to LG-R.

Disclaimer

None.

References

Balietti, M., Casoli, T., DiStefano, G., Giorgetti, B., Aicardi, G., & Fattoretti, P. (2010). Ketogenic diets: An historical antiepileptic therapy with promising potentialities for the ageing brain. *Ageing Research Reviews*, *9*(3), 273–279. https://doi.org/10.1016/j.arr.2010.02.003.

Bostock, E. C. S., Kirkby, K. C., & Taylor, B. V. M. (2017). The current status of the ketogenic diet in psychiatry. *Frontiers in Psychiatry*, *8*, 43. https://doi.org/10.3389/fpsyt.2017.00043.

Brandt, C., Nozadze, M., Heuchert, N., Rattka, M., & Löscher, W. (2010). Disease-modifying effects of phenobarbital and the NKCC1 inhibitor bumetanide in the pilocarpine model of temporal lobe epilepsy. *Journal of Neuroscience*, *30*(25), 8602–8612. https://doi.org/10.152 jneurosci 3/.0633-10.2010.

Choi, Y. J., Jeon, S. M., & Shin, S. (2020). Impact of a ketogenic diet on metabolic parameters in patients with obesity or overweight and with or without type 2 diabetes: A meta-analysis of randomized controlled trials. *Nutrients*, *12*(7), 2005. https://doi.org/10.3390/nu12072005.

Delpire, E., & Gagnon, K. B. (2018). Water homeostasis and cell volume maintenance and regulation. *Current Topics in Membranes*, *81*, 3–52. https://doi.org/10.1016/bs.ctm.2018.08.001.

Fedorovich, S. V., Voronina, P. P., & Wassem, T. V. (2018). Ketogenic diet *versus* ketoacidosis: What determines the influence of ketone bodies on neurons? *Neuronal Regeneration Research*, *13*(12), 2060–2063. https://doi.org/10.4103/1673-5374.241442.

Gómez-Lira, G., Mendoza-Torreblanca, J. G., & Granados-Rojas, L. (2011). Ketogenic diet does not change NKCC1 and KCC2 expression in rat hippocampus. *Epilepsy Research*, *96*(1–2), 166–171. https://doi.org/10.1016/j.eplepsyres.2011.05.017.

Granados-Rojas, L., Jerónimo-Cruz, K., Juárez-Zepeda, T. E., Tapia-Rodríguez, M., Tovar, A. R., Rodríguez-Jurado, R., Carmona-Aparicio, L., Cárdenas-Rodríguez, N., Coballase-Urrutia, E., Ruíz-García, M., & Durán, P. (2020). Ketogenic diet provided during three months increases KCC2 expression but not NKCC1 in the rat dentate gyrus. *Frontiers in Neuroscience*, *14*, 673. https://doi.org/10.3389/fnins.2020.00673.

Gulati, S. (2018). Dietary therapies: emerging paradigms in therapy of drug resistant epilepsy in children. *The Indian Journal of Pediatrics*, *85*(11), 1000–1005. https://doi.org/10.1007/s12098-018-2779-9.

Hami, J., Kheradmand, H., & Haghir, H. (2014). Sex differences and laterality of insulin receptor distribution in developing rat hippocampus: an immunohistochemical study. *Journal of Molecular Neuroscience*, *54*(1), 100–108. https://doi.org/10.1007/s12031-014-0255-1.

Kahle, K. T., Staley, K. J., Nahed, B. V., Gamba, G., Hebert, S. C., Lifton, R. P., & Mount, D. B. (2008). Roles of the cation-chloride cotransporters in neurological disease. *Nature Clinical Practice Neurology*, *4*(9), 490–503. https://doi.org/10.1038/ncpneuro0883.

Kahle, K. T., Rinehart, J., & Lifton, R. P. (2010). Phosphoregulation of the Na-K-2Cl and K-Cl cotransporters by the WNK kinases. *Biochimica et Biophysica Acta*, *1802*(12), 1150–158. https://doi.org/10.1016/j.bbadis.2010.07.009.

Kaila, K., Price, T. J., Payne, J. A., Puskarjov, M., & Voipio, J. (2014). Cation-chloride cotransporters in neuronal development, plasticity and disease. *Nature Reviews Neuroscience*, *15*(10), 637–654. https://doi.org/10.1038/nrn3819.

Kang, H. C., Lee, Y. M., Kim, H. D., Lee, J. S., & Slama, A. (2007). Safe and effective use of the ketogenic diet in children with epilepsy and mitochondrial respiratory chain complex defects. *Epilepsia*, *48*(1), 82–88. https://doi.org/10.1111/j.1528-1167.2006.00906.x.

Koumangoye, R., Bastarache, L., & Delpire, E. (2021). NKCC1: Newly found as a human disease-causing ion transporter. *Function*, *2*(1), zqaa028. https://doi.org/10.1093/function/zqaa028.

Kwon, Y. S., Jeong, S. W., Kim, D. W., Choi, E. S., & Son, B. K. (2008). Effects of the ketogenic diet on neurogenesis after kainic acid-induced seizures in mice. *Epilepsy Research*, *78*(2–3), 186–194. https://doi.org/10.1016/j.eplepsyres.2007.11.010.

McDonald, T. J. W., & Cervenka, M. C. (2018). Ketogenic diets for neurological disorders. *Neurotherapeutics*, *15*(4), 1018–1031. https://doi.org/10.1007/s13311-018-0666-8.

Meor, A. N. F., & Zhang, J. (2020). Role of the cation-chloride-cotransporters in cardiovascular disease. *Cells*, *9*(10), 2293. https://doi.org/10.3390/cells9102293.

Moser, M. B., & Moser, E. I. (1998). Functional differentiation in the hippocampus. *Hippocampus*, *8*(6), 608–619. https://doi.org/10.1002/(SICI)1098-1063(1998)8:6<608::AID-HIPO3>3.0.CO;2-7.

Paoli, A. (2014). Ketogenic diet for obesity: Friend or foe? *International Journal of Environmental Research and Public Health*, *11*(2), 2092–2107. https://doi.org/10.3390/ijerph110202092.

Paxinos, G., & Watson, C. 2007. *The rat brain in stereotaxic coordinates*. London: Academic Press.

Plotti, F., Terranova, C., Luvero, D., Bartolone, M., Messina, G., Feole, L., Cianci, S., Scaletta, G., Marchetti, C., Donato, V. D., Fagotti, V, Scambia, G., Panici, P. B., & Angioli, R. (2020). Diet and chemotherapy: The effects of fasting and ketogenic diet on cancer treatment. *Chemotherapy*, *65*(3–4), 77–84. https://doi.org/10.1159/000510839.

Qu, C., Keijer, J., Adjobo-Hermans, M. J. W., van de Wal, M., Schirris, T., van Karnebeek, C., Pan, Y., & Koopman, W. J. H. (2021). The ketogenic diet as a therapeutic intervention strategy in mitochondrial disease. *International Journal of Biochemistry and Cell Biology*, *138*, 106050. https://doi.org/10.1016/j.biocel.2021.106050.

Seyfried, T. N., Marsh, J., Shelton, L. M., Huysentruyt, L. C., & Mukherjee, P. (2012). Is the restricted ketogenic diet a viable alternative to the standard of care for managing malignant brain cancer? *Epilepsy Research*, *100*(3), 310–326. https://doi.org/10.1016/j.eplepsyres.2011.06.017.

Stafstrom, C. E., Wang, C., & Jensen, F. E. (1999). Electrophysiological observations in hippocampal slices from rats treated with the ketogenic diet. *Developmental Neuroscience*, *21*(3–5), 393-399. https://doi.org/10.1159/000017389.

Stafstrom, C. E., & Rho, J. M. (2012). The ketogenic diet as a treatment paradigm for diverse neurological disorders. *Frontiers in Pharmacology*, *3*, 59. https://doi.org/10.3389/fphar.2012.00059.

Strange, B. A., Witter, M. P., Lein, E. S., & Moser, E. I. (2014). Functional organization of the hippocampal longitudinal axis. *Nature Reviews Neuroscience*, *15*(10), 655–669. https://doi.org/10.1038/nrn3785.

Sun, D., Mei, L., & Xiong W. (2023). Dorsal dentate gyrus, a key regulator for mood and psychiatric disorders. *Biological Psychiatry*, *93*(12), 1071–1080. https://doi.org/10.1016/j.biopsych.2023.01.005.

Wang, S., Ding, Y., Ding, X. Y., Liu, Z. R., Shen, C. H., Jin, B., Guo, Y., Wang, S., & Ding, M. P. (2016). Effectiveness of ketogenic diet in pentylenetetrazol-induced and kindling rats as well as its potential mechanisms. *Neuroscience Letter*, *614*, 1–6. https://doi.org/10.1016/j.neulet.2015.12.058.

West, M. J., Slomianka, L., & Gundersen, H. J. G. (1991). Unbiased stereological estimation on the total number of neurons in the subdivisions of the rat hippocampus using the optical fractionator. *Anatomical Record*, *231*(4), 482–497. https://doi.org/10.1002/ar.1092310411.

Wheless, J. W. 2004. History of the ketogenic diet. In: *Epilepsy and the ketogenic diet*, edited by Stafstrom, C. & Rho, J. M., 31-50. Totowa: Humana Press Inc. https://doi.org/10.1007/978-1-59259-808-3_2.

Wheless, J. W. (2008). History of the ketogenic diet. *Epilepsia*, *49*(s8), 3–5. https://doi.org/10.1111/j.1528-1167.2008.01821.x.

Xie, Y., Chang, S., Zhao, C., Wang, F., Liu, S., Wang, J., Delpire, E., Ye, S., & Guo, J. (2020). Structures and an activation mechanism of human potassium-chloride cotransporters. *Science Advances*, *6*(50), eabc5883. https://doi.org/10.1126/sciadv.abc5883.

Index

#

2-deoxy-D-glucose, 11
4-aminobutyrate aminotransferase, 63, 65

α

α-secretase, 46, 47

β

β-catenin, 1, 8, 9, 15
β-hydroxybutyrate (BHB), 2, 3, 4, 19, 20, 24, 29, 31, 32, 34, 42, 44, 49, 50, 52, 53, 59, 67, 90, 94, 95, 97, 98, 99, 100, 109, 110, 111, 120, 126, 127, 128, 132, 135, 139, 142, 144, 145, 148, 149, 153
β-hydroxybutyric acid (BHB), 2, 3, 4, 29, 31, 32, 34, 42, 44, 49, 50, 52, 53, 94, 95, 97, 98, 99, 100, 109, 110, 111, 120, 126, 127, 128, 132, 135
β-oxidation, 3, 100, 134

A

acetoacetate, 4, 24, 29, 31, 44, 94, 95, 120, 125, 126, 128, 144
acetone, 29, 31, 44, 95, 97, 98, 100, 125, 144
acetylation, 4, 58, 99, 111
acetyl-CoA, 4, 5, 31, 97, 98, 99, 100, 107, 125, 128, 132
acid-sensing channels (ASIC), 2, 13
adenosine diphosphate (ADP), 2, 6, 7, 11
adenosine monophosphate-activated protein kinase (AMPK), 2, 7, 8, 14, 16

adenosine triphosphate (ATP), 1, 2, 4, 5, 6, 7, 8, 11, 14, 15, 18, 19, 21, 30, 31, 32, 42, 44, 46, 48, 52, 53, 94, 100, 101, 107, 120, 123, 131, 132, 134
aerobic fermentation, 102
agmatine, 10, 15, 81
Alzheimer's disease (AD), 42, 43, 44, 46, 47, 48, 49, 50, 51, 52, 54, 55
Amantadine, 28
amino acid metabolism, 21, 91, 103, 110, 116
amyloid plaques, 44, 46, 47, 48
amyloid β-peptide, 43, 56
amyloidogenic pathway, 46, 47
antibiotics, 13
anticholinergic medications, 28
anti-inflammatory effects, 44, 75, 94, 132
anti-inflammatory properties, 3, 15
anxiety, vii, 25, 51, 64, 75, 76, 77, 78, 79, 80, 82, 83, 85, 87, 88, 90, 153
apolipoprotein E, 42, 54, 57
aspartate, 10, 11, 66, 71, 120, 128, 131
astrocytes, 10, 47, 67, 90, 119, 124, 127, 128, 129, 130, 131, 133, 134, 140
astrocytoma, 110
autism, vii, 62, 64, 66, 71, 72, 73, 74, 79, 80, 81, 82, 83, 85, 86, 87, 88, 89, 91, 152
autism spectrum disorder (ASD), vii, 62, 64, 66, 71, 72, 73, 74, 79, 80, 82, 83, 85, 86, 87, 88, 89, 152
autism treatment evaluation test (ATEC), 62, 73
autonomic dysfunction, 25

B

Bcl-2-associated death-promotor (Bad) protein, 8
Beckomberga rating scale, 70
betaine gamma-aminobutyric acid transporter type 1 (BGT-1), 62
bipolar disorder, vii, 62, 64, 66, 78, 79, 80, 81, 83, 84, 85, 88, 91
bipolar I, 78
bipolar II, 78
body weight, 34, 142, 145, 148
bradykinesia, 25
BTBR mice, 74, 89

C

calbindin, 12, 86
calcium (Ca^{2+}), 2, 4, 5, 6, 9, 10, 11, 12, 18, 19, 52, 53, 62, 65, 72, 83, 124, 134
calcium signals, 134
caloric restriction, 67, 82, 95, 97, 99, 102, 108, 110, 130, 139
cancer, vii, 24, 93, 94, 95, 96, 97, 98, 99, 100, 101, 102, 103, 104, 105, 106, 107, 108, 109, 110, 111, 112, 113, 114, 115, 116, 124, 126, 135, 144, 156
cancer prevention, 94, 95, 99
carbohydrate, 1, 8, 23, 24, 29, 33, 34, 43, 44, 45, 64, 83, 86, 91, 111, 121, 123, 139, 143, 146
carnitine palmitoyltransferase I, 120, 131
caspase 3, 12
cell cycle, 96, 97, 107, 109
cell death, 2, 5, 9, 12, 47, 52, 96, 104, 105
childhood autism rating scale (CARS), 62, 73
chloride (Cl), 10, 62, 65, 67, 120, 128, 142, 143, 144, 146, 152, 155, 156
chloride importer, 152
chronic demyelination, 133
chronic inflammation, 48, 55, 103, 104
classic ketogenic diet (CKD), 24, 29
c-Myc, 9
cognitive functions, 43, 44
cornus ammonis, 142, 150, 152
corticotropin, 75
cortisol, 10, 75
counting frame, 147
cyclin D, 9, 17

D

demyelinating diseases, 133
dentate gyrus, 9, 11, 14, 67, 84, 128, 142, 145, 146, 147, 148, 149, 150, 151, 152, 153, 155, 156
depression, vii, 25, 51, 62, 64, 66, 74, 75, 76, 78, 79, 82, 85, 86, 87, 89, 90, 91, 153
direct pathway, 26
dizocilpine, 64, 71
DNA methylation, 94, 98, 104, 123
dopamine, 10, 15, 26, 27, 28, 30, 35, 67, 75, 89
dorsal region, 142, 147, 151

E

enzyme, 5, 7, 10, 31, 46, 62, 63, 65, 98, 100, 102, 129
ependymal cells, 134
epigenetic, 94, 95, 98, 99, 115
epilepsy, vii, 1, 2, 3, 5, 11, 12, 15, 16, 17, 18, 19, 20, 24, 32, 38, 44, 51, 57, 58, 61, 64, 67, 72, 82, 85, 95, 114, 121, 126, 127, 136, 139, 141, 143, 145, 152, 153, 154, 155, 156
euthymia, 75, 91

F

fasting, 24, 61, 64, 95, 97, 99, 107, 121, 122, 123, 130, 132, 143, 145, 156
fat, vii, 23, 30, 34, 38, 43, 61, 64, 93, 95, 99, 108, 121, 123, 138, 139, 140, 141, 144, 146
fatty acids, 3, 5, 8, 12, 18, 29, 31, 44, 50, 100, 115, 128, 130, 132, 133, 140, 144

G

GABA levels, 62, 66, 67, 69, 70, 72, 77, 78, 79, 80, 84, 85, 90
GABA transporters, 65
GABA type A receptors, 10
GABA/creatine, 78
$GABA_A$, 2, 10, 11, 62, 63, 65, 67, 68, 69, 72, 75, 77, 78, 80, 81, 82, 83, 85, 86, 88, 90
$GABA_A$ α, 62, 63, 85
$GABA_A$ α1, 62, 85
$GABA_A$ α2, 62
$GABA_A$ α3, 62
$GABA_A$ α4, 63
$GABA_A$ α5, 63
$GABA_A$ α6, 63
$GABA_A$ β, 63, 75
$GABA_A$ β1, 63
$GABA_A$ β2, 63
$GABA_A$ β3, 63, 75
$GABA_A$ γ, 63, 69, 75
$GABA_A$ γ1, 63
$GABA_A$ γ2, 63, 69, 75
$GABA_A$ γ3, 63
$GABA_A$ δ, 63, 75
$GABA_A$ ε, 63
$GABA_A$ θ, 63
$GABA_A$ π, 63
$GABA_A$-benzodiazepine receptor, 75
$GABA_B$, 63, 65, 69, 72, 79, 83, 88
GABABR1, 63, 65, 69, 72, 78
GABABR1a, 63, 65, 69
GABABR1b, 63, 65
GABABR2, 63, 65, 69, 72
$GABA_C$, 63, 65
GABAergic interneurons, 65, 69, 70, 72
GABAergic system, 62, 66, 68, 70, 78, 79, 152
GABA-T, 63, 65, 67
GAD65, 63, 65, 67, 68, 72
GAD67, 63, 65, 67, 68, 69, 72, 84, 91
galanin, 11
gamma-aminobutyric acid (GABA), 2, 7, 10, 11, 13, 14, 15, 62, 63, 64, 65, 66, 67, 68, 69, 70, 72, 75, 76, 77, 78, 79, 80, 81, 82, 83, 84, 85, 87, 88, 89, 90, 120, 121, 126, 128, 134, 135, 141, 142, 144, 152
gamma-aminobutyric acid transporter (GAT), 62, 63, 64, 65, 68, 69
GAT-1, 63, 65, 68, 69
GAT-2, 63, 65
GAT-3, 64, 65
generalized anxiety disorder, 62, 66, 76, 77, 79
glia, 60, 65, 119, 121, 122, 123, 124, 126, 128, 129, 130, 131, 132, 133, 134, 135, 136, 137, 138, 139
glioblastoma, 108
globus pallidus, 24, 26
glucose, 3, 7, 8, 11, 15, 16, 29, 33, 42, 43, 44, 45, 51, 52, 53, 61, 73, 100, 101, 102, 107, 108, 109, 110, 111, 114, 119, 120, 121, 123, 124, 126, 127, 129, 130, 131, 132, 134, 139, 140, 142, 144, 145, 148, 149
glutamate, 10, 11, 13, 14, 15, 16, 17, 65, 66, 67, 72, 75, 78, 81, 82, 83, 86, 87, 89, 103, 120, 121, 124, 127, 128, 130, 131, 132, 134, 135, 138
glutamate decarboxylase, 10, 11, 87, 128
glutamic acid decarboxylase, 62, 63, 65, 82, 84, 90
glutamic acid decarboxylase enzyme (GAD), 62, 63, 65
glutaminase, 120, 131, 132
glutamine, 8, 10, 11, 78, 86, 90, 103, 127, 128, 130, 131, 132, 134
glycemic index treatment, 24, 30
glycolysis, 8, 9, 11, 14, 15, 44, 51, 52, 100, 101, 102, 107, 123, 129, 130, 131, 132, 133
granule layer, 9, 142, 148, 150, 151, 152
gut microbiota, 4, 12, 15, 16, 17, 18, 76, 104

H

hallmarks of tumor, 100
hepatocytes, 8, 98, 100, 130

high-fat, 11, 134, 138, 143
hilus layers, 147, 150, 153
hippocampal epileptogenesis, 11
hippocampal formation, 68, 72, 81, 152, 153
hippocampus, 4, 5, 8, 9, 10, 11, 13, 15, 18, 20, 21, 32, 39, 52, 66, 67, 69, 78, 81, 91, 124, 150, 152, 153, 155, 156
histone modifications, 98, 99
hormones, 10, 11, 75
hydroxymethylglutaril-CoA synthase, 98
hyperpolarization, 1, 2, 7, 65, 121
hypomanic episode, 78
hyporexia, 76
hypothalamus, 13, 134, 138

I

immunohistochemistry, 146
indirect pathway, 26, 27
inflammasome, 12, 20, 32, 49, 50, 58, 94, 105, 106, 109, 110, 115
inflammation, 4, 12, 14, 16, 41, 42, 43, 48, 50, 55, 57, 58, 60, 94, 96, 103, 104, 105, 107, 109, 114, 115, 116, 123, 126
inhibitory neurons, 65, 69
inner mitochondrial membrane, 52
insulin secretion, 109
interleukin 1b, 12
intracellular chloride concentration, 142, 144, 152
ion channels, 5, 6, 16, 21
ionic homeostasis, 11

K

K^+/Cl^- cation-chloride cotransporter, 64, 67
K^+/Cl^- cation-chloride cotransporter 2 (KCC2), 64, 67, 84, 120, 128, 137, 143, 144, 145, 152, 155
kainate, 9, 17
K_{ATP} channels, 1, 2, 6, 7, 8, 9, 14, 17, 19
KCC2 cotransporter, 145, 152

ketone bodies, vii, 2, 3, 6, 7, 17, 20, 21, 24, 29, 31, 32, 42, 44, 53, 58, 60, 61, 64, 66, 83, 84, 94, 95, 97, 99, 100, 102, 107, 108, 110, 112, 114, 115, 119, 120, 121, 123, 125, 128, 137, 144, 154
ketone bodies (KB), vii, 2, 3, 4, 5, 6, 7, 8, 10, 11, 12, 13, 17, 20, 21, 24, 29, 30, 31, 32, 42, 44, 45, 46, 50, 52, 53, 54, 58, 60, 61, 64, 66, 83, 84, 94, 95, 97, 99, 100, 102, 107, 108, 110, 112, 114, 115, 119, 120, 121, 123, 125, 126, 127, 128, 129, 130, 133, 134, 135,136, 137, 138, 140, 144, 154
ketosis, vii, 3, 11, 15, 21, 24, 29, 33, 35, 36, 37, 38, 43, 59, 60, 61, 64, 71, 79, 80, 81, 91, 93, 95, 97, 102, 112, 119, 120, 121, 122, 123, 126, 127, 128, 129, 130, 132, 134, 135, 138, 139, 153

L

lactate, 2, 13, 19, 101, 107, 109, 114, 120, 129, 130, 131, 132, 133, 140
lactate dehydrogenase (LDH), 2, 13, 19, 120, 131
laterality, 142, 147, 153, 155
leptin, 10, 19, 20
levodopa, 28
Lewy bodies, 25
limbic system, 44, 153
lithium, 79, 90, 91
long-term safety, 36

M

major depressive disorder, 75, 76, 77, 89
manic episode, 78
medium-chain triglyceride diet (MCTD), 24, 29
metabolic oxidation, 120
metabolism, 4, 5, 6, 8, 11, 12, 13, 14, 15, 16, 28, 29, 30, 33, 38, 44, 50, 51, 52, 56, 57, 59, 60, 79, 84, 86, 96, 99, 100, 101, 102, 103, 107, 108, 111, 114, 115, 116,

119, 121, 126, 127, 129, 130, 135, 136, 137, 138, 139, 140, 143
microglia, 47, 48, 49, 50, 56, 57, 59, 124, 132, 135, 137, 138
mitochondria, 2, 4, 6, 12, 14, 18, 20, 42, 51, 52, 53, 59, 97, 100, 101, 102, 107, 110, 125, 131, 132, 144
mitochondrial ATP-sensitive potassium channels, 52
mitochondrial biogenesis, 3, 4, 14, 30, 32, 53
mitochondrial complex I and IV, 5
mitochondrial dysfunction, 5, 8, 15, 26, 30, 43, 51, 81, 102, 108, 116, 133, 144
mitochondrial respiratory chain, 46, 155
MK-801, 64, 71
molecular layer, 11, 143, 150, 152
molecular mechanisms, vii, 2, 96, 97, 105
monogenetic, 54
mood, 33, 77, 78, 79, 81, 83, 90, 110, 156
Müller cells, 134, 139
multiple sclerosis, 50, 133
myelin, 124, 133, 139, 140

N

Na$^+$/K$^+$-ATPase pump, 11
neurodegenerative diseases, vii, 29, 36, 44, 46, 51, 126
neurofibrillary tangles, 47, 51
neuroglia, 48, 119, 120, 121, 122, 123, 126, 129, 135
neuroinflammation, 12, 23, 26, 30, 32, 48, 51, 58, 60, 140
neuronal death, 8, 9, 12, 26, 29, 47, 51, 130
neuron-astrocyte complex, 127
neuropeptide Y, 11
neuroprotection, 2, 12, 18, 20, 29, 32, 53, 59, 135, 139
neurotoxicity, 12, 17, 38, 44
neurotransmission, 62, 65, 66, 67, 77, 80, 88, 124, 142, 144, 152
neurotransmitter, 4, 5, 10, 12, 13, 14, 65, 66, 67, 75, 121, 130, 135, 136, 138, 141, 144

neurotransmitter production, 13, 130
neurotrophins, 46, 50
NF-kB, 120, 132
N-glycolylneuraminic acid, 104
NKCC1, 84, 137, 141, 142, 143, 144, 145, 146, 147, 148, 149, 150, 151, 152, 153, 154, 155
NKCC1 cotransporter, 142, 144, 145, 150, 152, 153
NLR family pyrin domain containing 3 (NLRP3), 12, 20, 42, 49, 50, 58, 94, 105, 106, 107, 109, 110, 115
normal diet, 34, 143, 145, 146, 149, 151, 152
nuclear factor κB, 94, 104

O

oligodendrocyte precursors, 120, 132
oligodendrocytes, 119, 124, 133
oncogenes, 98, 101
optical fractionator, 142, 147, 156
oxaloacetate, 10, 11, 126, 128
oxidative stress, 2, 4, 5, 6, 14, 17, 18, 19, 20, 23, 24, 30, 41, 43, 51, 56, 57, 73, 75, 107, 111, 126, 127

P

P20/N40 gating, 71
P2Y1 receptor, 134
pentylenetetrazole, 9
polygenetic, 54
Porsolt Test, 76
positive and negative symptom scale, 64, 70
postural instability, 25
pro-inflammatory cytokines, 12, 32, 48, 106
protein, vii, 2, 3, 5, 8, 10, 13, 14, 16, 20, 24, 25, 30, 42, 43, 44, 46, 47, 49, 50, 51, 52, 55, 56, 57, 58, 59, 60, 61, 64, 65, 68, 69, 76, 82, 84, 87, 94, 96, 103, 105, 108, 109, 141, 143, 144, 146, 150
PV-immunoreactive interneurons, 72

R

rat, 14, 15, 19, 20, 21, 34, 35, 38, 39, 66, 67, 79, 83, 84, 90, 111, 137, 139, 142, 146, 152, 155, 156
reactive oxygen species (ROS), 2, 3, 4, 5, 6, 9, 12, 17, 24, 30, 32, 42, 45, 46, 48, 51, 52, 53, 54, 58, 76, 107, 134
reduced glutathione, 5, 129
rigidity, 25, 28

S

schizophrenia, vii, 51, 62, 64, 66, 67, 68, 69, 70, 71, 79, 80, 81, 82, 83, 84, 85, 86, 87, 88, 89, 90, 91, 152
Schwann cells, 121, 133
side effects, 4, 28, 29, 35, 36
Sprague-Dawley, 80, 145
stereo investigator 9 software, 147
stereological system, 147
stereology, 142, 147, 151
substantia nigra, 24, 25, 26, 27
succinic semialdehyde, 64, 65

T

tanycytes, 134, 136, 138
Tau protein, 43, 44, 47

the long-term use of alcohol, 104
tremors, 25, 33
tricarboxylic acid cycle, 10, 66, 94, 102
tripartite synapse, 127, 129
tuberin protein, 3, 10
tumor microenvironment, 101
two-pore domain K^+ channels (K2P), 2, 8, 12, 16

U

uncoupling proteins (UCPs), 3, 5, 12, 52, 53
urea cycle, 103, 110

V

valproic acid (VPA), 64, 74, 80, 82, 90
ventral region, 143, 147, 150, 151, 153
vesicular GABA transporter, 65
vesicular gamma-aminobutyric acid transporter (VGAT), 64, 65
vesicular glutamate transporters, 10

W

Warburg effect, 94, 100, 101, 107, 110
Wnt, 1, 8, 9, 10, 14, 15, 16, 17, 18, 19, 20
Wnt3a, 8, 9